Fit for Rugby

REX HAZELDINE and TOM McNAB

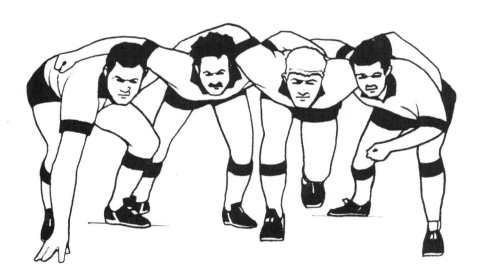

THE KINGSWOOD PRESS

First published in Great Britain in 1991
by The Kingswood Press
an imprint of Methuen London
Michelin House, 81 Fulham Road, London sw3 6rb

Copyright © 1991 Rex Hazeldine and Tom McNab

A CIP catalogue record for this book
is available from the British Library
ISBN 0 413 66010 9

Photoset by Rowland Phototypesetting Ltd
Bury St Edmunds, Suffolk
Printed in Great Britain
by BPCC Hazell Books, Paulton and Aylesbury

Contents

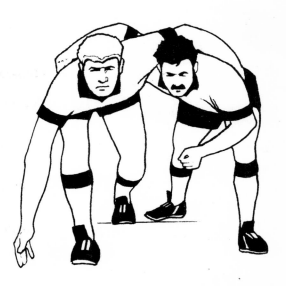

Acknowledgements

There are many people we need to thank for their help in preparing and developing this book: in particular, Barney Kenney, Alan Foster and Jim McKenna, the other RFU fitness advisers, who have made an enormous contribution to fitness preparation for rugby football; Geoff Cooke, Roger Uttley, John Elliott, Kevin Murphy, Dr Ben Gilfeather, Dr Terry Crystal, Dick Best, Mike Slemen, Graham Smith and Eric Lewis, the senior England management teams, for their constant support of our fitness advisory work with the England squads; Don Rutherford, the RFU's technical director, for all his help, not least for agreeing to write the foreword to this book; and also to Chalkie White, Tony Biscombe, Keith Bonser, and Des Diamond, the RFU divisional technical administrators, and to Alan Black, the national promotions officer, for their co-operation and assistance.

We must also thank Jim Holmyard and his predecessor, Rosie Mayes, for co-ordinating the England rugby fitness advisory project; their help with the fitness testing programme has been invaluable. We are grateful also for the interest and encouragement shown by Captain Mike Pearey RN, whose term of office as president of the Rugby Football Union coincided with the development of this book, and also Penny Rowe, Bill Hazeldine and Michael Hazeldine for their help in preparing for production the manuscript of the book. Finally, rugby football is essentially about players and it has been our privilege to work with the talented and committed members of the England squad, without whose supportive presence on and off the field this book might not have been written.

Rex Hazeldine, Tom McNab

The photographs on the cover and inside the book are reproduced by kind permission of Colorsport. The publishers are also much indebted to the skill, patience and enthusiasm of Roger Towers for all his original drawings.

Foreword

DON RUTHERFORD

Technical Director, Rugby Football Union

In persuading the Rugby Football Union to invite Tom McNab, a former national athletics coach, to act as the catalyst for our National Fitness Programme, I was totally confident he would make an impact. Some of the players in 1986–87, when the programme began, were enthusiastic converts immediately; others were sceptics with the deepest conviction born of the fact that everything had come to them without expending much effort.

Former England coaches, such as Dick Greenwood and Martin Green, had manfully planted the early seeds but it was Tom of the Dunstablians fourth team who added the fertiliser. Tom introduced the England squad to Judy Oakes and Mike Winch, both British shot-putt champions. Judy and Mike were steeped in weight training and track work and the sight of Judy power-cleaning 200lb at Bisham Abbey left most of the England forwards absolutely gobsmacked. Most did not even know how to lift weights safely, let alone understand the differences between training for strength or power.

Tom McNab is some salesman, believe me, and has a wonderful Glaswegian patter which has painted in the minds of players some strikingly sharp pictures of what is needed to optimise their natural ability. Once the selling was well under way, Rex Hazeldine, an RFU senior coach, was grafted on to the operation as the organiser of our fitness-testing programme. We are particularly grateful to Loughborough University, where the programme is monitored and to Rex, who is the director of the Centre for Coaching and Recreation in the University and is also the director of coaching for rugby football there. Their programmes have now been personalised to meet the needs of each individual and his position on the field. The whole programme is supported through the generosity of the Sports Council and the National Coaching Foundation.

The rugby that England have produced in the last three years has been quite outstanding and owes much to Rex and Tom, but in particular to the enthusiasm and dedication of the players. As Tom always says, 'I cannot get you fit, only you can do that; what I can do is show you how'. I know the principles illustrated in this book do work but you must take the trouble to understand them and then put them into action.

The game of the future will demand rugby players who are athletically trained, and this will result in a far more free-flowing, running and handling game.

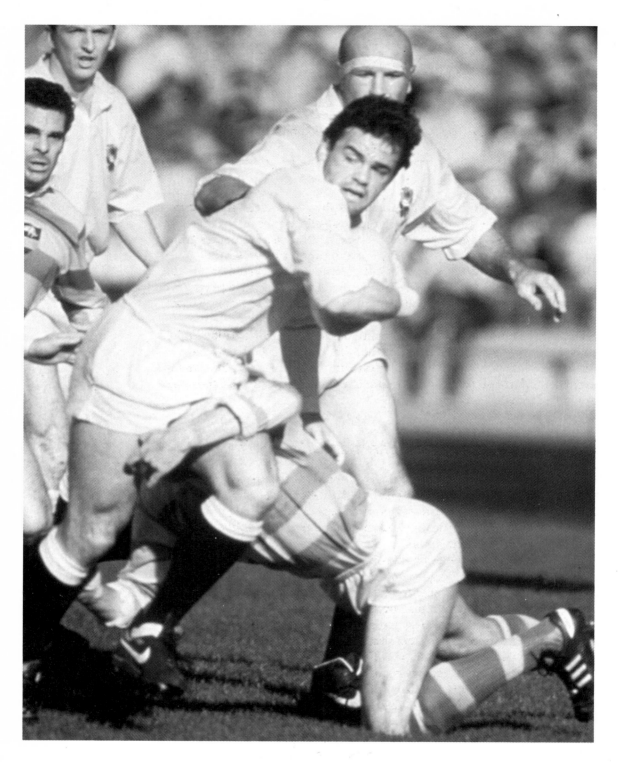

England captain Will Carling is half-held in the tackle
by his Argentinian opponent, and begins to look round for support.

Chapter 1

Getting the Basics Right

'You can't fire a cannon from a canoe'
(Anon)

This is a book about fitness for committed rugby players at all levels of the game. It combines the lessons of practical experience with the best teachings of modern sports science. Some of the material comes from other sports, athletics in particular. For the rugby player is an athlete, albeit a contact athlete. He must be committed to the game and must reflect on it. He must be physiologically and psychologically strong and he must be fit and fast and mobile, capable of running until hell freezes over.

Incidentally, the rapidly increasing numbers of women who play rugby must forgive us for referring throughout the book to players as male as if we believed that women had no serious part to play in the game. That is emphatically not our view: we hope that many women will read the book and be helped by it.

Fitness – the responsibility of the player

It was Abraham Lincoln who said that 'those who fail to prepare must prepare to fail'. Both skill development and fitness training are inter-dependent parts of modern rugby preparation. It is the degree to which a player prepares himself in these areas that ultimately determines his performance on the field of play.

The modern rugby player has become as different from his counterpart of a quarter of a century ago as athletes in any other branch of modern sport. Simply to turn up at a couple of loosely organised club training sessions each week, then to play on a Saturday, is not sufficient, even at junior club level. Rugby football, aided by catalysts such as the World Cup and league club rugby, is now coming into line with other major sports.

Fitness is the responsibility, not of the club but of the player himself. This does not mean that club sessions cannot have an impact on fitness. Rather it means that it is what a player does when he is on his own that determines his level of match-fitness. And in this sense, a rugby player is no different from a swimmer or a weight-lifter.

Of course, there are many who play rugby simply for recreation and who see no need to train or to attend club training sessions. These are players who turn up with their gear every Saturday afternoon, play their game, have a few beers and do nothing in the way of training until they play again a week later. This book is not addressed to them. We would, however, observe that a basic level of health-related fitness cannot be achieved simply by playing rugby or any other game once a week. Games do not develop fitness, rather they reflect it. Thus, there is a need even for the recreational player to swim or walk or run to meet the needs of general health.

Why be fit?

The essence of rugby is the ability to sustain high levels of skill at high speed over the full 80 minutes of a game. The aim of any fitness programme is to make this possible. Fitness, in effect, is the background against which skill can be achieved and maintained within the game.

However, it is often forgotten that fitness also enables skills to be developed in training sessions involving a large volume of high-quality activity. This relates particularly to endurance fitness, which is quite literally at the heart of any fitness programme.

The core of fitness lies in endurance, the ability to sustain high-quality effort, and thus produce whatever skills and techniques a player posses-ses over the whole of the game. The crisis-point in many games is towards the end of the first half and more often towards the end of the second half when fatigue begins to dull vision, errors begin to occur, tackles are missed. Endurance fitness enables players to retain the quality of their play in these crucial periods.

Of course, endurance is not the only element, although it is an important one, particularly for the forwards. Running speed is also critical, as rugby is essentially a running game. Similarly, strength, particularly upper body strength, is essential in tackling and mauling situations and in scrummaging.

One of the significant features of the period from 1986 onwards with the England team has been the lower incidence of injuries; and this correlates with the massive increase in fitness-levels which has been achieved during this period. Clearly, fitness cannot guarantee freedom from injury, but it does help considerably. The England team physiotherapist, Kevin Murphy, used his own measure, which he called his 'Vaseline count'. This related to the number of pots of Vaseline which he used on the insides of players' thighs before each game to minimise chafing. This dropped, within a year, with the increasing muscularity of players and consequent drop in body fat, from almost two pots a game to less than half a pot!

One element which has not been mentioned so far is natural fitness, the fitness which a player brings to the game independent of training. The greatest players almost invariably bring a high level of natural fitness to the game. As an example, Rory Underwood long-jumped almost 7m as a schoolboy; and in an athletics fitness test, in a backward two-handed shot throw, he achieved 17m 26cm, a world-class performance. Indeed, top-class players bring to their sport a high level of athleticism and are, in effect, 80 per cent of the way there when they come to the game. It is, however, what they do with the final 20 per cent that counts at international level, and players with lower levels of natural fitness can often catch up with more talented players simply by committing themselves to their fitness training.

Time management

The aim of any training programme, whether it relates to technical development or fitness, is to get the maximum effect in the minimum possible time.

When the England team were first exposed to formal fitness regimes back in 1986 in preparation for the 1987 World Cup, the first aim was to make efficient use of their existing time. It was found that many players were failing to do this, that they were using long slow runs when they needed accelerative speed, that they were using high repetition weight training for strength when they needed heavier weights and lower repetitions. This was, in essence, the misuse of time by the employment of the wrong kinds of training. Other players were failing to use available time before the start or at the end of club sessions or at lunch-time to enhance their fitness. Our aim is to minimise the amount of time in training by using every possible minute of training time to maximum effect.

The specificity of training

Training is specific in two ways. The first lies in physiological specificity, in that different types of training produce different results. A simple example lies in sustained low-pace runs over, say, a distance of 5,000m. This produces endurance but no speed or strength and, if a player does too much of it, it can even reduce power and flexibility. Conversely, sprint training does nothing to develop endurance, though it clearly enhances running speed.

Table 1 Training

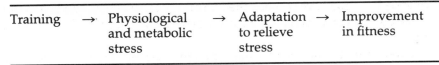

Training	→	Physiological and metabolic stress	→	Adaptation to relieve stress	→	Improvement in fitness

The second kind of specificity lies in positional specificity, in that different positions require different types of fitness. We will look at the detail of positional differences later, but it is clear that the fitness requirements of a prop are not the same as those of a full-back, simply because the game-demands of the two positions are of a totally different nature.

11

Training is essentially about adaptation, about the body's response to the stress of exercise. Exercise challenges the body, forcing it to respond in order to cope with the possibility of another challenge (Table 1). Thus the body's muscles, for example, adapt either by increasing their ability to take up oxygen, or in their ability to work at speed.

Muscle type

Broadly speaking, there are two main types of muscle-fibre, fast-twitch and slow-twitch, and everyone possesses a balance of these two types.

Fast-twitch fibres are capable of explosive contractions but have little endurance capacity. In contrast, slow-twitch fibres have poor explosive qualities but have high oxygen-carrying capacities.

An international sprinter might, therefore, have an 80/20 balance in favour of fast-twitch fibres, while a marathon runner might have a similar balance in favour of slow-twitch fibres. In rugby terms, we are probably looking at fast-twitch athletes in the backs and half-backs; in the props and second row we may be looking at a 50/50 balance; and in the back row and hooker probably at 60/40 in favour of fast-twitch.

The heart is a muscle of a totally different nature, in the sense that it is not subject to skeletal control and it does not conform to the fast-twitch/slow-twitch formula. It is, however, capable of adapting in the same way as the voluntary muscles, in that it can increase both in its endurance and in the strength of its contraction, according to the type of training which it is given.

Warm-up and cool-down

Warm-up

Before every training session, practice game or match it is essential to warm up thoroughly in order to provide the body with a period of adjustment from rest to exercise. Warm-up improves a player's physical efficiency by raising the heart, metabolic and respiratory rates. If demands are made gradually on the circulatory and respiratory systems no sudden or extreme discomfort is felt. Warm-up is also designed to improve performance and reduce the risk of injury by mobilising the player mentally as well as physically.

By raising both the general body and deep muscle temperatures and by stretching the muscle and connective tissue (which, together with the increased temperature, improves the elasticity of the muscle) the possibility of muscle tears, ligament strains and muscle-soreness is reduced. Warm-ups can, of course, contain the rehearsal skill-patterns and ball-work which will occur in the following practice session or match. The effects of warm-up will ultimately wear off, so players should warm up in a track-suit and keep warm during breaks in training. Here are some simple guidelines:

1 There should be a whole-body warm-up which progressively raises body temperature and gradually increases the heart rate; for example, jogging or work on an exercise bicycle or a rowing machine.

2 The muscles and connective tissue should be carefully stretched by working systematically through the main muscles and joints.

3 The routine should be a combination of intensity and duration but without undue fatigue.

4 There should be no time-lag, especially in cold conditions, between warm-up and training or competition.

Most players usually appreciate the value of warm-up but often seem unaware of the equally important need to cool down after training.

Cool-down can be defined as exercises performed immediately after training to provide the body with a period of adjustment from exercise to rest. When the period of exertion is over, many adaptations have to be made during the process of recovery before the body returns to normal.

These recovery processes, such as the removal of muscle and blood lactic acid, are helped by an active rather than a passive activity. This means a few minutes of jogging, walking and mild rhythmic-type muscular activity, gradually decreasing in intensity. Stretching should also be included during the cool-down period. Consequently, a cool-down routine will not only promote the removal of waste products but will also facilitate muscular relaxation and reduce muscle-soreness.

Game analysis

The analysis of the work-demands of athletic events is relatively easy because it is not that difficult to work out the oxygen requirements of running 5,000m in 14 minutes. A game such as rugby presents a much more complex problem, since the demands of each game and of each position are quite different. As an example, a winger or full-back might spend much of a game with almost nothing to do, a physiological demand of almost zero. A week later, the same players could be under intense pressure, sprinting and tackling with a work-demand ten times the amount of the previous week. The aim must be to prepare each player for the hardest game which he is likely to play at his level of performance.

A number of studies have shown that backs, on average, cover a total distance of about 4,000m and forwards between 5,000–6,000m, which means that forwards run about 20 to 30 per cent further than backs. We see, too, that the volume of running, particularly faster running, increases significantly from club to national level:

Table 2 Average yardage by level of game

	Jog	Sprint/stride	Total
Club	3,800	225	4,025
County	4,700	552	5,252
National	4,908	1,700	6,608

Wade Dooley, the great England lock, some years ago made the massive leap from junior club rugby to the national team. In his first international game he was exhausted at half-time, having made three times as many fast runs in the first half as he previously made in a whole game.

The big increase at international level, in fitness terms, is undoubtedly the pace of the game and the way in which that pace is sustained throughout the full 80 minutes. This is clearly the result of more than mere speed of foot and relates also to speed of thought. However, even speed of thought can be dulled by fatigue; and the longer fatigue can be withstood the more easily speed of thought can be maintained. Thus the need for endurance.

If we look, too, at the amount of time the ball is in play, we see that it is in play for only 25 per cent of the time and that most of the continuous action lasts for less than 20 seconds. For example, in the 1991 Wales v England match at Cardiff Arms Park the ball was in play for 22 minutes 35 seconds. There were 132 activity cycles in the game of the following durations:

Table 3a Activity cycles

Duration (seconds)	Number of cycles
0–4	38
5–8	35
9–14	25
15–19	16
20–24	10
25–29	6
30–40	0
Above 40	2
TOTAL	132

The results were similar later in the season, when England played Ireland at Lansdowne Road. The ball was in play in this match for 26 minutes 56 seconds. There were 126 activity cycles of the following durations:

Table 3b Activity cycles

Duration (seconds)	Number of cycles
0–4	36
5–8	23
9–14	26
15–19	16
20–24	8
25–29	8
30–40	6
Above 40	3
TOTAL	126

A study undertaken in France tried to assess the work-demands placed on each position during a match by analysing twenty-eight forwards and the same number of backs at the top level of French rugby. The results were recorded in some detail.

Under contact play the French included wrestling, shoving, jumping and tackling. Running requirements were considered under headings of jogging, fast runs and sprints. For the forwards, in addition to the work involved in an average of 40 scrums, 55 line-outs and 70 rucks and mauls, running speeds involved jogging most frequently, with jogging three times as frequent as fast running. For the forwards, running never occurs in isolation; rather it happens immediately before and after contact play with nearly all sprints limited to a distance of 30m with jogging rarely exceeding 60m.

For the backs, the play was characterised by periods of inactivity interspersed with brief, but extremely intense, bursts of activity. In each match, a number of play sequences could be observed involving a succession of runs at various speeds and duration, following closely upon one another and often accompanied by a fairly hard collision. As an example, for a centre, a play sequence lasting 55 seconds could consist of 3 sprints and 3 fast runs, 2 tackles and three pauses of 5 seconds. The centres seemed to carry out most of the tackles.

Fast runs were the prerogative of full-backs; for other positions the average run (including sprinting and fast running) was between 30 and 40m.

The analysis of the positional match-demands naturally indicated the need for separate fitness training for forwards and backs. The study suggested, for example, that some of the training for forwards should consist of a series of activity-sequences with exercises or be given over to contact play combined with running. Within their fitness programme, the threequarters should be training as sprinters based on rugby running, which means, for example, running while avoiding tackles, running and experiencing impacts, running sequences with speed and direction changes, and sprinting, including passing the ball.

The French study shows the difficulty in analysing any game, particularly one like rugby. Indeed, this type of evaluation can be accused of stating the obvious, but it does supplement the little objective information on match-demands which we possess.

It certainly highlights the massive positional variations in the game compared with soccer and hockey, in which all the players perform roughly the same skills and experience similar physiological demands. No team game, except possibly American Football, shows such a variation of demands as rugby.

When match analysts indicate how long the ball is in play, and that the typical length of an interval of work can be quite short, this is a one-dimensional view of the game. A maul, for example, lasting 25 seconds, can leave the forwards limp with fatigue and may be followed by a set scrum. The game also has a body-contact element which is not easily measurable. Here we come up against the term 'body hardness', a term which most players will recognise. This hardness has little to do with strength or endurance and can only be secured by match play or by team practices involving body contact.

Positional requirements

There are, of course, common fitness demands for every player but, as discussed, rugby probably incorporates the most marked inter-positional differences in fitness requirements. What follows in this section is an attempt to identify some of the qualities needed in different positions. In planning a fitness programme, emphasis should be placed always on developing positional qualities so that schedules not only meet the individual needs of a player and the overall demands of the game but also specific positional fitness requirements.

Rather than cover every position, we have divided the team into the following groups, containing positions with common requirements:

1 Props and locks
2 Back row and hooker
3 Half-backs
4 Backs.

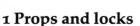

1 Props and locks

a *Running/endurance fitness.* This will help them to carry out support running after scrums and line-outs, to be there at breakdowns, to be involved in running and handling, to help maintain the continuity of the attack, to cover in defence.

b *Strength and power.* They must develop leg power for driving forward in scrum, ruck and maul, for line-out jumping (in the case of locks), for running into the opposition with the ball. They need strength in the lower back and shoulders, particularly in the scrum, and strength in the upper arms and chest to enable strong binding in scrums, line-outs, rucks and mauls.

c *Speed.* They need to develop, particularly, acceleration away from scrums, line-outs, rucks and mauls.

d *Flexibility.* They must develop an adequate range of movement, especially in the shoulder and hip joints, and generally good all-round flexibility.

2 Back row and hooker

a *Running/endurance fitness.* This is essential for the back row who endure more running than anyone in the team – over 5,000m in most games including support running, attacking running with the ball, and covering in defence.

b *Strength and power.* They need to develop leg power for driving forward in scrum, ruck and maul (the push of the back row is vital in the scrum); back, shoulder and arm strength for scrum-binding and in line-outs, ruck and maul, and for wrestling and ripping the ball away in tackle and maul situations.

c *Speed*. They must develop speed of reaction and leg speed (in the case of the hooker); acceleration in order to be first to the breakdown, first to the ball, speed to get into position and support the ball carrier, and speed for attacking running with the ball.

d *Flexibility*. The hooker needs to develop a range of movement in shoulder, spine and hip, and all must acquire generally good all-round flexibility.

3 Half-backs

a *Running/endurance fitness*. They need to be always in position to receive the ball from forwards; as well as developing their support running, attacking running with the ball, and covering in defence.

b *Strength and power*. These they must develop in order to drive into the opposition and 'stay on their feet', and to absorb contact.

c *Speed*. They need to develop acceleration off the mark from scrum, line-out, ruck and maul, to make a break, and to support the ball carrier.

d *Flexibility*. They need to develop a good all-round range of movement.

4 Backs

a *Running/endurance fitness*. Much of the running for backs consists of sprinting with changes of pace; for example, the full-back moves from three-quarter pace to full pace as he enters the line, the wing needs to control and vary pace, and will need to undertake a certain amount of support running and covering in defence.

b *Strength and power*. These qualities they must develop in order to drive into the opposition and 'stay on their feet', to absorb contact from the opposition, and to make a tackle.

c *Speed*. They need to develop acceleration and speed off the mark, pure running speed, change of pace and direction, speed to chase kicks, and speed to cover in defence.

d *Flexibility*. They need to develop a good all-round range of movement, particularly in the hips.

Chapter 2

The Training Programme

'Luck is the meeting of preparation and opportunity'
(Anon)

Fitness training for rugby football is complex and involves an endless search for the link between training and performance. This is done by structuring a training programme which can be adapted to the needs of the player and the team, and which can be integrated with the specific demands of particular matches.

The approach to adopt, known in athletics as periodisation, is to organise the training period into a number of divisions in the pursuit of basic training objectives. This is done:

1 To prepare the player for optimal improvement in performance
2 To prepare him to meet the total match-demands during the season
3 To prepare him for significant matches during the season
4 When appropriate, to help him recover from injury, illness or a particularly stressful match or training period.

The starting point to all this is an evaluation of the fitness requirements of rugby football. In order to clarify the various components which affect fitness for the game it is useful to develop a model of physical fitness for rugby football. This enables the fitness elements which make up the training programme to be identified.

Table 4 Model of physical fitness for rugby football

Body composition		Nutrition and diet		Rest and relaxation
Flexibility		**Fitness for rugby**		Aerobic endurance
Speed	Agility	Strength	Power	Contact fitness

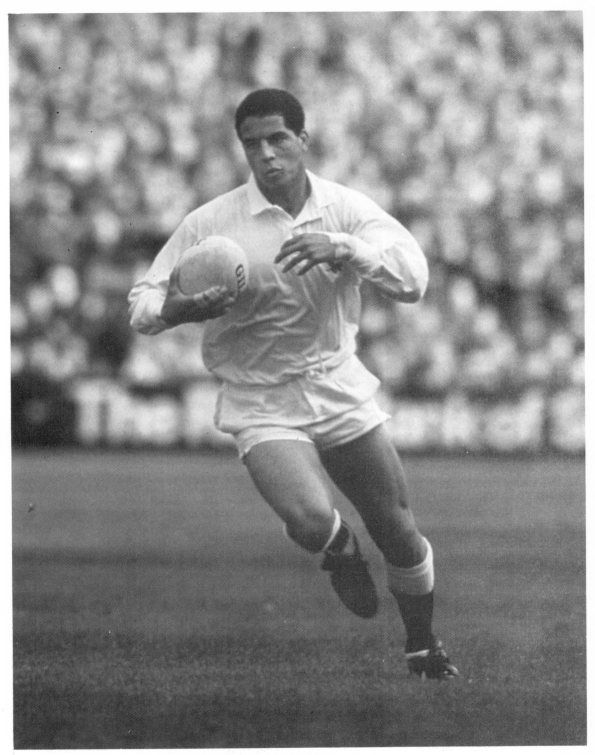

Jeremy Guscott sets off on another
beautifully balanced run.

Then take this evaluation a stage further, by adding the individual and positional requirements for the players.

Table 5 Positional requirements

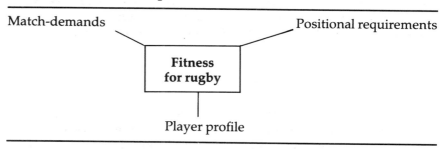

Match-demands

We know that a game of rugby lasts for 80 minutes, of which on average the ball is in play for 25 minutes, the remainder (55 minutes) consisting of stoppages of one sort or another; from a physical point of view those are rest periods. The interval of work on average is 10 seconds and the interval of rest is 25 seconds. There are about 125 sequences of play during a match. So the player needs to have a capacity to produce a sequence of high energy bursts punctuated with moments of rest. There is also, of course, a contact element within the game creating a need for contact fitness.

Rugby football, like many other games from a fitness point of view, is a multiple sprint sport with sequences of high energy bursts but it also has specific and almost unique fitness requirements. Therefore it is important, when structuring a training programme, that these specific requirements are fully met in order that busy players are not subjected to irrelevant, time-consuming training sessions.

Positional requirements

The inter-positional differences in rugby football are probably greater than in most other team games and those were described in some detail in Chapter 1. Thus, though they are both involved in the same game, the demands on the tight-head prop are quite different from those on the wing. Relating this to track and field athletics, the prop can be compared in some ways to a discus thrower whereas the winger might well be compared to a sprinter. In spite of this, many clubs provide almost identical fitness training sessions and programmes for all players in the team, an outdated approach which fails to meet the different positional fitness needs of each player.

In a similar way, players will vary as individuals in their fitness requirements. There will be age differences which need to be taken into consideration. Certain players will be lacking in leg power or upper body strength; they will need to develop better accelerative speed or be more flexible. Each player will have a unique fitness profile and any good fitness programme should be individualised and personalised.

Structure

Training should be structured to provide stages or divisions in the total programme which vary in duration and in the nature and intensity of the training prescription practised at each stage. To be on a sound physiological basis, training should be planned on a year-long cyclical process, but one which is also part of a long-term progression of training. It is important that the structure meets the particular training and match requirements of a team so a year-long cycle incorporating one season is appropriate. But this cycle can be extended, as is shown in the England squad's fitness training schedule for the 1991 World Cup, which embraces an 18-month programme building up to the start of the competition at Twickenham (Table 6).

This plan shows the time-scale in weeks; the international, divisional and club commitments of the players; the squad training and fitness testing sessions; the various training stages and training phases (specifying the area of fitness to be developed); the training unit (specifying the details of each training session, to be prescribed after each testing session); the changes in volume of training and the timings to achieve peak levels of fitness. The World Cup plan tries to show how all these factors need to be considered and successfully integrated into a total fitness training schedule. Although there will always be particular objectives – whether preparing for the World Cup or for a single season – a training programme should also have longer-term objectives for a player, looking forward over two or even three seasons of development.

At the outset, planning is based on a simple cycle of training which includes preparation, competition and recuperation stages.

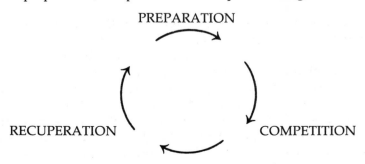

PREPARATION

RECUPERATION   COMPETITION

Table 6 England Squad – Fitness Training Schedule for the 1991 World Cup

MONTH	MAY				JUNE					JULY				AUGUST				SEPTEMBER					OCTOBER				NOVEMBER				DECEMBER				
A WEEKS TO GO	74	73	72	71	70	69	68	67	66	65	64	63	62	61	60	59	58	57	56	55	54	53	52	51	50	49	48	47	46	45	44	43	42	41	40
B SATURDAYS	5	12	19	26	2	9	16	23	30	7	14	21	28	4	11	18	25	1	8	15	22	29	6	13	20	27	3	10	17	24	1	8	15	22	29
C INTERNATIONAL + TOURS	ITALY																										ARGENTINA								
D PILKINGTON CUP, DIVISIONAL + CLUB LEAGUE MATCHES																				LEAGUE MATCH (1)	BARBARIANS		LEAGUE MATCH (2)	LEAGUE MATCH (3)	LEAGUE MATCH (4)	LEAGUE MATCH (5)		LEAGUE MATCH (6)	LEAGUE MATCH (7)	PG 3RD ROUND	DIVISIONAL CHAMPIONSHIP				
E SQUAD TRAINING SESSIONS & TESTING																SQUAD TRAINING ON TOUR			SQUAD TRAINING (7/8th)					SQUAD TRAINING (28th)											
F PERFORMANCE PEAK, (T) = FITNESS TESTING	75% / 50% / 25%				(T)							ARGENTINA TOUR						(T)									[3]								
G TRAINING STAGE	[1]													[2]																					
H TRAINING PHASE	REST				ENDURANCE AND STRENGTH BASE					INTERVAL RUNNING, RUNNING DRILLS & PLYOMETRICS + STRENGTH								HIGH QUALITY SPEED WORK AND POWER DEVELOPMENT					SHORT RECOVERY WORK AND POSITION SPECIFIC POWER				MAINTENANCE				"ACTIVE" REST				
I TRAINING UNIT	1.				2.					1.	2.	3.		1.	2.	3.		2.	1.	2.			1.	2.			2.				1.				
J FITNESS TRAINING VOLUME	75% / 50% / 25%																																		

	JANUARY				FEBRUARY				MARCH					APRIL				MAY				JUNE				JULY				AUGUST					SEPTEMBER			
Week	39	38	37	36	35	34	33	32	31	30	29	28	27	26	25	24	23	22	21	20	19	18	17	16	15	14	13	12	11	10	9	8	7	6	5	4	3	2	1
Date	5	12	19	26	2	9	16	23	2	9	16	23	30	6	13	20	27	4	11	18	25	1	8	15	22	29	6	13	20	27	3	10	17	24	31	7	14	21	28

Events:

- LANZAROTE (3rd–6th JAN) — (T)
- LEAGUE MATCH (8)
- WALES (B. vSPAIN)
- PC/4TH ROUND
- LEAGUE MATCH (9)
- SQUAD TRAINING (10th)
- SCOTLAND (B. vITALY)
- PC. QTR. FINAL
- SQUAD TRAINING (24th)
- IRELAND E (IRELAND E)
- LEAGUE MATCH (10)
- SQUAD TRAINING (10th)
- FRANCE (FRANCE E)
- PC. SEMI. FINAL
- LEAGUE MATCH (11)
- LEAGUE MATCH (12)
- PC. FINAL
- TOUR
- SQUAD TRAINING ON TOUR
- PRACTICE GAME (1)
- PRACTICE GAME (2)
- PRACTICE GAME (3)
- WORLD CUP ASSEMBLY
- (T) markers in May/June and August

Training phases:

[4]				[5]			[6]	
FIVE NATIONS PREPARATION	MAINTENANCE	REST	MAINTENANCE	REST	ENDURANCE/INTERVAL RUNNING (←STRENGTH)	HIGH QUALITY SPEED WORK AND POWER DEVELOPMENT	SHORT RECOVERY WORK AND POSITION SPECIFIC POWER	'GAME RELATED' FITNESS WORK	TAPER PERIOD

Prepared by Rex Hazeldine and Jim Holmyard. England Rugby Fitness Advisory Project. Supported by the Sports Council.

Preparation

The preparation stage can be divided into two distinct phases:

1 *Out-of-season*: Here the emphasis is on general training with a relatively high volume of work in order to develop a fitness base. On this should be built the specialised and more game-specific training which will follow.

2 *Pre-season*: Now the training is specifically related to the demands of rugby football and the player's level of development.

1 *Out-of-season*: Today most players of a good standard recognise the value of maintaining some degree of physical fitness out of season. In fact this is a vital, if not the most vital, stage in the whole training programme. Out of season, the player should maintain and develop certain levels and types of fitness which provide a logical base for the more intensive pre-season training. The out-of-season phase is also an ideal time for working on recovery from injury and on limitations and weaknesses from the previous season. Another important element is endurance training, described in Chapter 3.

Time is available out of season for the type of continuous training, which is effective in developing a sound 'aerobic base', the crucial foundation needed for other forms of training to follow. There should be concentration on continuous sub-maximal exercise, such as long continuous running, cycling or swimming with training high in volume but low in intensity. More severe methods of training such as Fartlek or interval training can be used at a later stage.

As the player is not involved in a match schedule, it is also a good time for strength training. The early schedule should be a general one with emphasis on the main muscle groups, for example, squats, bench press, clean, or high pull to provide a 'strength base' for the more specific strength work later. Flexibility work should be included and not neglected at any stage in the programme, particularly when the player is involved in strength work.

2 *Pre-season phase*: Based on sound and progressive out-of-season training, the pre-season work should be designed to bring the player to a high level of fitness for the start of the season. There is a gradual change of emphasis during this phase from quantity to quality of training. The intensity of the endurance training can be increased by progressively introducing more high-quality Fartlek and interval training. Training schedules will be introduced which aim to improve muscular endurance, anaerobic capacity and speed. The main objective in the pre-season strength programme is preparation to meet the demands of the sport, so within strength training there will be a change of emphasis from general strength work to more specialised strength exercises. There is also the crucial need to develop power, so training methods such as plyometrics can be used effectively at this stage.

It is worth pointing out that it is quite usual to note lower fitness levels during the middle part of the season, when crucial matches are being played, than in the early part. Indeed, it is not unusual to see a rugby player's fitness decrease over the season. One of the reasons for this is a hurried and inadequate preparation period with no solid foundation on which to build the high levels of specialised and game-related fitness needed for crucial matches in the middle or later part of the season.

Competition

Physical fitness is reversible, though it takes less time to maintain an improved fitness level than it does to achieve it. Too many players abandon serious training once the season starts because of lack of time, match-demands or a false assumption that matches themselves will develop the necessary fitness. The player who has trained seriously and progressively through the preparation stage faces the prospect of regression during a long season unless an appropriate fitness programme is maintained. In fact, maintenance is one of the key words for the competitive stage.

Endurance fitness can be maintained on one or two sessions per week. Long easy-paced runs on a Sunday, for example, can be used as light but active recovery from the heavy demands of matches or they can form the basis of a long warm-up prior to a practice or fitness session.

Anaerobic capacity needs to be maintained and even increased during the season so regular anaerobic training (for example, shuttle running or short interval work) needs to be done regularly at least once a week. In the strength area, the aim is to maintain levels of specialised strength, to develop new levels of competitive-based strength and power, and to help prevention of injury. One or two sessions a week on strength training should be sufficient.

Recuperation

Most players understandably see the end of a long season as the start of a lengthy period of rest and relaxation away from the game. Full recovery and recuperation, both physical and mental, from the rigours of the season are essential in order to provide maximum potential for the next cycle of training.

In fact, this recuperation phase is not a gap in the training programme but an essential link between the competitive and preparation phases. It should involve a gradual reduction in all forms of training, rather than a sudden withdrawal, and a transition to lighter, more relaxing activities, such as tennis, squash or swimming. These must be chosen, with no element of compulsion; they will also have important psychological effects and, above all, provide a continuance of physical activity which will help to maintain a reasonable level of fitness.

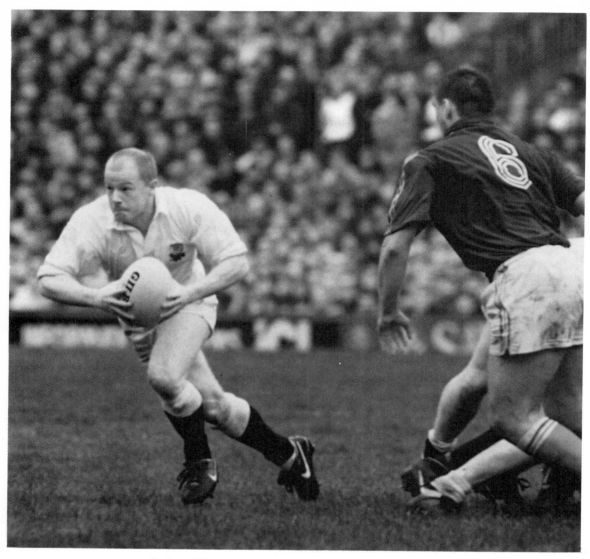

Bath and England's Richard Hill breaks from the base of the scrum
in the 1991 Five Nations decider against France at Twickenham.

Chapter 3

Endurance

'Fatigue makes cowards of us all'
(Vince Lombardi)

Endurance training is, quite literally, at the heart of rugby, because without endurance it is impossible to retain a high quality of technical skill and mental focus throughout the game. Similarly, without a good level of endurance, it is difficult to acquire skills in training simply because of recurring fatigue.

The rugby player requires different types of endurance. To last the 80 minutes of the game, to recover between intervals of play, to possess 'runnability' and maintain a high work rate he needs good 'aerobic endurance', that is, the process of taking in, transporting and using oxygen to provide energy in the muscles.

The player also needs 'muscular endurance', that is, the capacity of the muscles to endure the continuous performance of localised activity, such as working with the arms and driving forward in a maul. He also needs a good 'anaerobic capacity' because rugby football produces repeated bursts of energy over short periods of time called 'multiple sprint activity'.

We will look at each of these qualities and the appropriate training in turn.

Aerobic endurance

The lungs, heart and blood vessels act as a supply system providing the muscles with necessary fuels and oxygen and carrying away waste products, such as carbon dioxide and lactic acid. Thus, the cardio-respiratory system in the rugby player needs to be developed to match the demands of the muscles which it supplies and cleanses. Aerobic capacity or 'maximum oxygen uptake', known by the abbreviation $\dot{V}O_2max$, is the maximum volume of oxygen which can be used per minute by a player. It is measured in litres/minutes but as there is variation in body size between players, it is usually reported per kilogram of body weight and is a good indicator of a player's endurance fitness.

Playing the game once a week does not develop endurance, rather it reflects it. This means that endurance, like all other factors of fitness, has to be developed outside the game itself. This does not mean that games and club practices cannot make a significant impact and these practices are outlined in Chapter 7. However, the aim must be for the player to bring a good level of endurance to his club practices, thus making it easier for the club coach to reach what he wishes to improve – the individual techniques and the team-skills of his players.

Endurance training follows precisely the same principles as all other forms of conditioning: it uses 'progressive overload', thus stimulating the body through the challenge of training to adapt by improving the capacity and the efficiency of the cardio-respiratory system.

The National Coaching Foundation's Multi-stage Fitness Test is described in Chapter 9 – a progressive shuttle-run test used by the England team to predict maximum oxygen uptake and therefore estimate endurance capacity. The progressive shuttle-run test should, ideally, be used as the starting point in any endurance programme, which should begin in early June after a period of 'active rest'.

The concept of 'active rest' was described more fully in Chapter 2 but here it is important to observe that rugby players should be pursuing endurance programmes throughout the year as a matter of general health, quite independently of the game. Thus, we would expect some light jogging during the period of 'active rest'. Similarly, we would expect a recreational player, with no specific rugby fitness requirement, to undertake this level of endurance activity simply as part of his basic fitness routines.

Endurance is probably as 'natural' a quality as sprinting and there are many examples of long-retired distance runners, men who have pursued no training for many years, being tested on treadmills and being found to have retained high levels of endurance. Our experience is that the backs, being lean and light, tend to have naturally high endurance levels and that it does not take much work to bring them up to acceptable levels of 60ml/kg × minute (see Chapter 9). The forwards, on the other hand, are 20–30kg heavier, and even at international level often start at the early 50ml/kg × minute level, not much better than many recreational players. Our experience shows that improvements of 10 per cent to 15 per cent are possible, using modern training methods; and we must bear in mind also improvements in body-fat percentages which will affect this value.

There are three basic methods of improving endurance fitness:

1 Long continuous running
2 Fartlek training
3 Interval training

1 *Long continuous running*: This is the foundation of the training programme. It is essentially aerobic, which means 'with use of oxygen', but in simpler terms means a level of effort at which oxygen uptake and energy output are in balance. In contrast, in sprinting, which is an anaerobic activity, the body uses other energy systems, such as glycolysis, to provide energy rapidly, with oxygen used after the sprint in order to facilitate recovery.

Long continuous running is the platform upon which the more severe and more specific types of endurance training (Fartlek and interval training) can be built. It is essentially the 'getting fit to train' type of endurance work. Before it is initiated in early June, the $\dot{V}O_2$max fitness test can be taken. Alternatively, there are tests such as the Cooper Test which aims to discover how far a player can run in 12 minutes and predict $\dot{V}O_2$max. These tests provide a bench-mark against which future improvements can be measured.

It is useful during training to be able to measure the heart rate as it gives a good indication of the intensity of effort. This can be done by taking the pulse, usually the radial pulse. To do this three fingers should be placed on the underside of the wrist in line with the base of the thumbs. Using a watch or stop-watch the number of beats per 15 seconds is counted then multiplied by 4 to give an estimate of heart rate per minute.

The long continuous runs should involve running at 'talking pace' at a distance of between 3 to 5 miles, 2 or 3 times a week, preferably on grass. These runs should be made over defined routes so that improvements can be logged. As the running becomes easier the distance should be increased while simultaneously trying to reduce the time. A player might start with an average of an 8-minute/mile pace over 2 miles. Six weeks later he might be running 5 miles at an average of a 7-minute/mile pace. Another possibility is to begin with a steady pace and run from a particular point for a specified length of time, say, 20 minutes. The distance run can then be increased while the time remains approximately the same.

It is essential that appropriate running shoes should be worn and this relates particularly to forwards. When we consider that forces of three times the body weight will be recorded on each stride and that in a 5-mile run there will be close on 10,000 strides, the need for correct footwear is clear. There are some excellent features involved in the design of modern road shoes which are as far from the running shoes of old as a modern fibreglass vaulting pole is from the old alloy type of the 1950s.

During the first long continuous running period, the aim should be to develop mileage, rather than increase speed. Thus a first week's mileage might be 10 miles and by the end of June this might be 20 miles. By this time the multi-stage shuttle-run test score might have gone from 11.2 to 12.2 and the resting pulse rate from 68 to 63 beats per minute. The body has, in effect, made some adaptations and we are now ready to go further.

Again, mileage can now rise marginally and the pace increased. This means that the player now goes beyond 'talking pace' to a level where the pulse is in the 150–170 beats per minute. This can easily be checked as described earlier.

2 *Fartlek training*: Fartlek is a Swedish word meaning 'speed play'. The player usually determines the length and timing of the intermittent changes in pace but it should be planned precisely to create overload situations with appropriate recovery phases. The forced entry into periods of anaerobic work and consequently oxygen debt during the fast pace demands repayment during the following phase of easy running. This acts as a stimulus for the improvement of maximum oxygen uptake

and speed of recovery, two very necessary qualities for a rugby player.
A typical Fartlek session consists of

Warm-up and stretching
Easy running   5 minutes
Half pace   5 minutes
Easy running   2 minutes
A series of fast strides 200m × 6 interspersed with 2 minutes easy
   jogging
Easy running   2 minutes
A series of uphill sprints 50m × 6 with jog-back recoveries
Cool-down (easy jogging) and flexibility work

3 *Interval training*: Interval training is a more formal version of Fartlek. It consists of running a specified number of distances, which for rugby players would be between 150m and 400m in a given time at about 80 per cent effort level with short walk-back recoveries or rest periods of about 2 minutes. For this form of training it is best to work on an athletics track where the running surface is good and the distances can be measured accurately. Each interval training session will vary according to the time of year and the fitness of the player by altering the length of the work interval, the pace of each run, the number of repetitions and the length of the rest intervals. A typical session during the out-of-season period could be 300 metres × 5 in 55 seconds with 2-minute walk-back recovery intervals between each run.

The heart-rate value, by checking the pulse counts, can be observed towards the end of the rest interval at, say, 1 minute 30 seconds and should have dropped below 130 beats per minute by the start of the next interval.

Anaerobic capacity

As we have already said, rugby involves bursts of high intensity effort such as sprinting which needs an enormous amount of energy very rapidly. The aerobic system cannot supply enough energy for sprint-type work so during those phases of the game when the player is working particularly hard a significant amount of energy is supplied from the anaerobic (without oxygen) systems. One of these energy systems, anaerobic glycolysis, can break down the stored carbohydrates (glycogen) to produce energy very rapidly, but one of the end products of the process is lactic acid which, as it builds up in the muscle, is one of the main causes of fatigue.

This build-up will tend to have two basic effects – 'enzyme inhibition', which slows down the whole process of glycolysis and thus the production of energy from this source; and 'mechanical impairment', where the actual process of muscular contraction is eventually interfered with, reducing the power output of the muscle.

Of course, all players experience this fatigue during the game, resulting from bouts of intense effort, and we need to provide training at the appropriate stage which helps the player to cope with the build-up of lactic acid in the muscle.

The type of training needed is 'short interval work' or 'shuttle running', which can be used to improve 'sprint explosiveness' and help the player recover from maximal or near-maximal bouts of work. There are a number of possible schedules which can be used:

1 Players can work for a set time interval of 40 seconds with an interval of rest of 20 seconds. The work interval can include sprinting to a line 10 or 15 metres away or wrestling for a ball – any number of appropriate rugby-related activities.

2 Players can work in pairs for a set time interval of 30 seconds, interspersed with 30 seconds rest. One player can sprint out to a line 10 metres away for 30 seconds, then rest while his partner runs. This can be modified by running to 10, then 15, then 20 metres during the work interval or using any appropriate rugby-related activity with or without the ball.

— can be incorporated with speed endurance training.

The player will now have reached a point where he has a good aerobic base and the beginnings through his Fartlek and interval training of a high aerobic capacity which will enable him to deal with the first club training sessions; also some early development of anaerobic capacity.

The emphasis must now be on pushing up the quality of the endurance sessions and developing other endurance qualities. There should be no big increase in mileage during August, for we must now consider the increase in specific training stress which has been added through club sessions and which will undoubtedly increase the intensity through the month.

Muscular endurance

This component of fitness overlaps with aerobic endurance and represents a player's ability to sustain continuous localised muscular activity. Such activity may make relatively small demands on the respiratory and circulatory systems before exhaustion sets in. Since muscular endurance is the ability to repeat muscular contraction over a period of time it is a quality which is vital to the rugby player and particularly to the forwards. The game requires players to work repeatedly the muscles of the arms and shoulders in wrestling for the ball in a maul situation or making a series of sprints or driving forward in a scrum. Indeed, there are countless instances of bouts of muscular effort by all players in the team.

— important but not vital for centre

The game requires different types and amounts of muscular activity. Consequently, different energy systems are brought into play and a player experiences fatigue when energy demand in the muscles is greater than the energy supplied. As previously indicated, if energy is required at a higher rate, glycolysis, an anaerobic system, uses glycogen stored in the muscle and converts it to energy. The other energy system, the aerobic system, can break down both the stored glycogen and fat.

There is a third energy system, the phosphocreatine system, which uses an energy-rich compound in the muscle, creatine phosphate, to produce energy. No oxygen is required for this system so it can be called anaerobic. This is used predominantly in the first few seconds of muscular activity as the creatine phosphate is there ready in the muscle.

A rugby player will use a combination of all of these energy systems and the degree of involvement of each system will depend on the nature and intensity of the work at the time. As work during the game is intermittent, with intervals of work and intervals of rest, the player will have time to recover from hard bouts of effort and is given the chance to replenish some of the energy stores during the rest intervals and remove the inhibiting waste products such as lactic acid.

The more often a muscle is trained to perform a certain movement over the same range, against the same resistance, and at the same frequency and speed as required during the game, then the less likely it is to become fatigued during play. The improvement is due to a number of factors:

1 the utilisation of oxygen by improving circulation and involving more blood capillaries, thus providing the working muscles with more oxygen and fuel

2 the involvement of more muscle fibres

3 speedier removal of the metabolic waste products of strenuous exercise.

Circuit training

One widely used and proven method of improving muscular endurance is circuit training. This can be organised on a club basis using normal equipment.

An example of each type of rugby circuit is described below but there are many possible variations and modifications in each category of circuit. The circuit should always be adapted to the needs of the players, to the situation, and to the facilities and equipment available.

Circuit training on the pitch

In pairs or in groups of 4
One minute at each station, 30 seconds rest while moving to the next station (Table 7)

1 *Sprints with walk-back recovery*: Sprint to a mark 30m away and then walk back to start.

2 *Clap-hand push-ups*: Front support position with arms shoulder width apart. Push up explosively, clap hands and then replace hands on floor. Both players working.

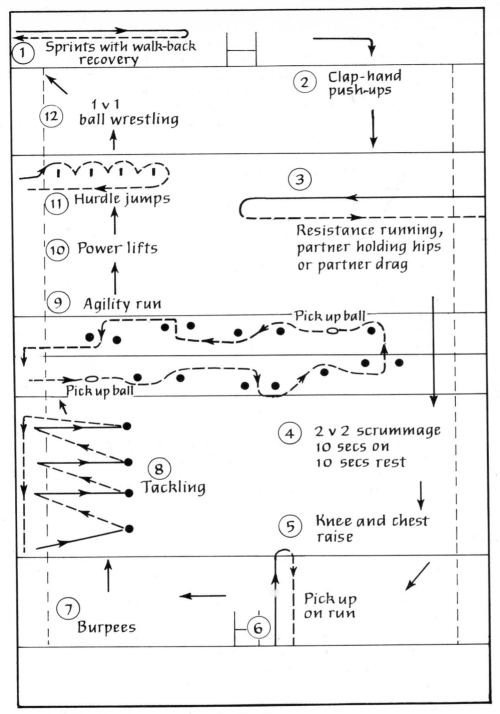

1. Sprints with walk-back recovery
2. Clap-hand push-ups
12. 1 v 1 ball wrestling
3. Resistance running, partner holding hips or partner drag
11. Hurdle jumps
10. Power lifts
9. Agility run
Pick up ball
Pick up ball
8. Tackling
4. 2 v 2 scrummage 10 secs on 10 secs rest
5. Knee and chest raise
7. Burpees
6. Pick up on run

Table 7 Circuit Training on the Pitch

3 *Resistance running, partner holding hips* (Fig 1) *or partner drag* (Fig 2): One partner takes hold of player's hips and sits back or puts his arms over one shoulder and under the arm on the other side and then the player runs 30m with this resistance from the partner. Change places to run back to the start.

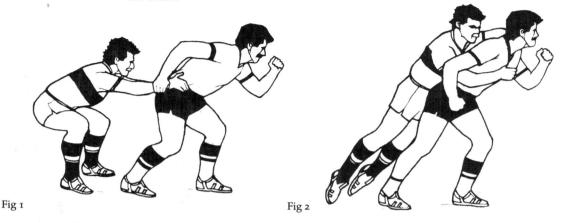

Fig 1   Fig 2

4 *2 v 2 scrummage* (Fig 3): Partners bind together and oppose the other two players in a two versus two scrummage. Work 10 seconds followed by 10 seconds rest; keep repeating same intervals of work and rest.

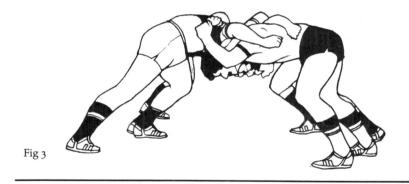

Fig 3

5 *Knee and chest raise* (Fig 4): Lie on back with knees bent and hands beside head, raise trunk and bring knees to chest at the same time. Both players working.

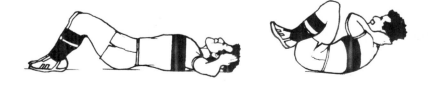

Fig 4

6 *Pick up on the run*: Partner rolls ball for player to run out and pick up, both players run to the 22-metre line. Player then rolls for partner to pick up and they both run back to try line.

7 *Burpees* (Fig 5): From a standing position, crouch to place hands on the floor in front of the feet, jump both feet back to crouch position and stand up. Repeat the complete movement rhythmically and continuously, both players working.

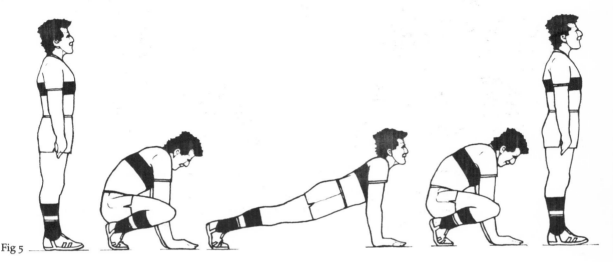

Fig 5

8 *Tackling* (Fig 6): From the 5-metre line, run and tackle the first bag; then quickly up and back to the 5-metre line, then run and tackle the second bag; continue tackling bags in rotation. All four players working. Assistants required to return bags to upright position.

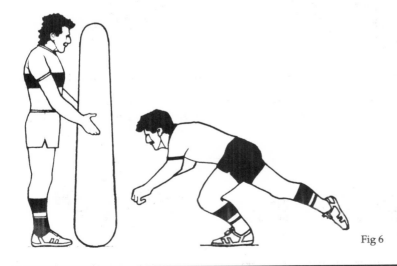

Fig 6

9 *Agility run with ball* (Fig 7): Players sprint from touchline, pick up ball, swerve through cones, side-step through two cones, swerve and side-step again, then put ball down. Then round the next cone, pick up a second ball, swerve then through two sets of cones back to start. Continue. All four players working.

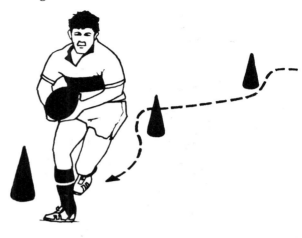

Fig 7

10 *Power lifts* (Fig 8): Player holds partner's legs securely in wheelbarrow position. Partner pushes explosively from floor and raises trunk with assistance from player. Change over at half-way (30 seconds).

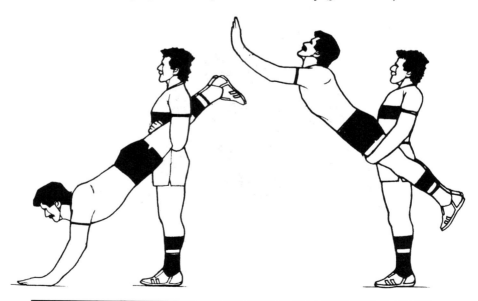

Fig 8

11 *Hurdle jumps* (Fig 9): Face first hurdle and begin by lowering the body, then jump explosively with both feet together and keeping knees high over hurdle. On landing, continue movements over remaining hurdles, concentrating on driving knees upwards and swinging arms forwards. All four players working, with walk-back recoveries.

Fig 9

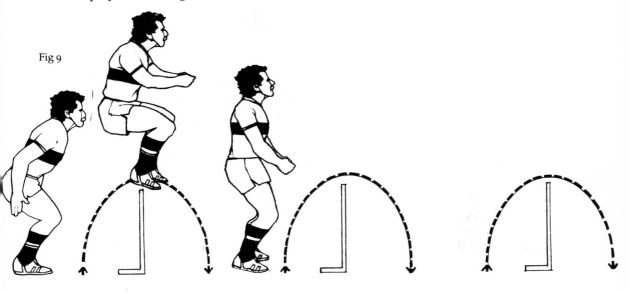

12 *Ball wrestling* (Fig 10): One ball between two players; player holds ball, partner tries to get hands on ball and 'rip it away' from player. 10 seconds work, 10 seconds rest. Change round the player in possession of the ball.

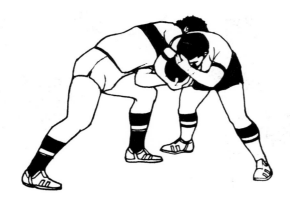

Fig 10

Rugby-specific circuit

Work in pairs. Work interval of 60 seconds
with an interval of rest of 30 seconds.

1 *Leg thrust* (Fig 11): Player lies on back with legs raised and held out
straight; partner holds on to player's feet and then presses player's knees
and hips into full flexion; player then presses and straightens legs against
the resistance which partner provides. Change half-way.

Fig 11

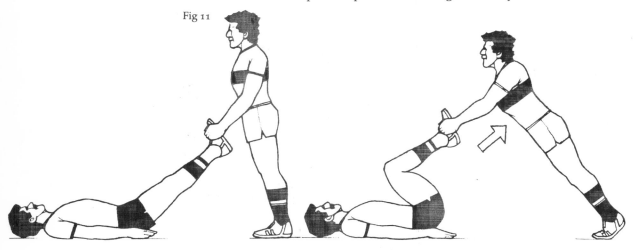

2 *Scrum-half pass*: Players stand 5m apart; the ball is placed on floor by first
player who, after passing to partner, runs back to a mark 5m away and
then returns to receive the pass from partner.

3 *Leg curl* (Fig 12): Both players adopt prone position on the floor and grip
a rugby ball between the feet; raise ball by flexing knees as far as possible.
Both players working.

Fig 12

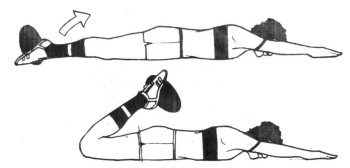

4 *Wrist roller* (Fig 13): Attach a suitable weight by a length of cord to a bar; by rotating the bar, roll up and unroll the weight with arms held out in front. Change half-way.

5 *Side-step* (Fig 14): Set out four cones as shown, run forward and side-step the cones in order; turn and side-step back to starting point; players alternate.

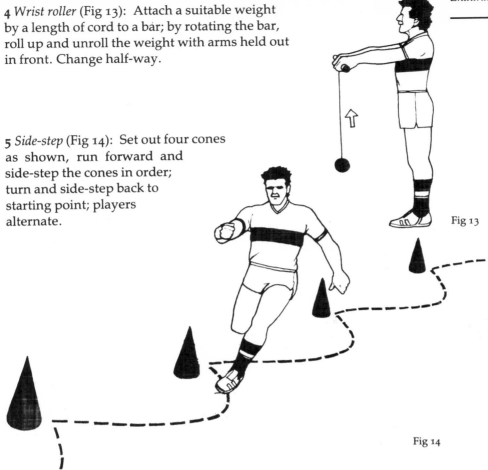

Fig 13

Fig 14

6 *Scrummaging* (Fig 15): Both players move forward from a distance of 3m and form one-man scrummage for 10 seconds; then return to the line for 10 seconds rest; and keep repeating the same intervals of work and rest.

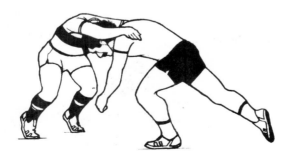

Fig 15

7 *Inter-passing*: Players move up and down a length of 20 to 30m, inter-passing with a distance of 3 to 5m between them.

8 *Bench crossover jumping* (Fig 16): Stand to one side of the end of a bench, facing along the length of the bench, jump diagonally across the bench and continue jumping from side to side down the bench, return by repeating the same movements. Players working together, one after the other.

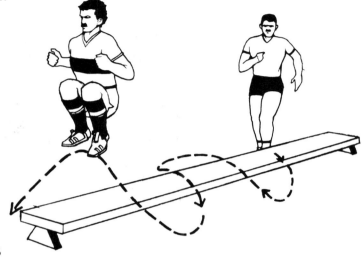

Fig 16

9 *Cradle carry* (Fig 17): Player carries partner in cradle position in front of his body over a distance of 10m; change places and partner carries player back to the start.

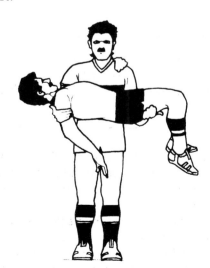

Fig 17

10 *Box rebound* (Fig 18): Partner stands on a five-section box or equivalent, holding a ball about half a metre above player's reach; player jumps to take ball, lands, then jumps immediately to return ball to partner on the box. Change half-way.

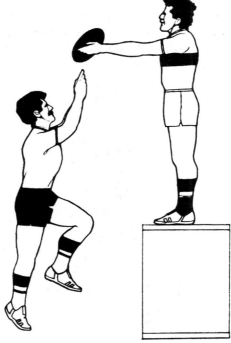

Fig 18

11 *Shuttle run*: From a starting line, a player sprints to a line 5m away and runs back; then to 10m and back; then to 15m and back; alternate with partner.

12 *Abdominal curl*: Both players lie on their backs with knees bent and hands beside the head, curl up and twist touching left knee with right elbow; then repeat, touching right with left elbow, continue alternating in this way. Both players working.

It is possible to have considerable variety in circuit training. For example, instead of a set of exercises at each station in rotation, it is possible for the players to move continuously round the circuit, using exercises which keep them moving forward.

The squad can be divided into pairs with one partner moving round the circuit in a set time, say 60 seconds, while the other partner rests. The partners then alternate. Or the circuit can be organised on the basis of five circuits each. As in all forms of fitness training it is important to have

Continuous circuit

41

appropriate work loads, intensities to suit each player's individual requirements, fitness levels and maturity.

The following is a possible plan for a continuous rugby activity circuit inside a gymnasium or sports hall (Table 8).

1 Vault over the buck
2 Double-footed jumps over a bench, working forwards
3 Run and jump on to a box; then jump to a second box
4 Two forward rolls on mats, working forward
5 Sprint between skittles
6 Run and jump on to a box; then jump to a second and to a third box, placed appropriate distances apart
7 A through-vault over horse
8 Spring jump between two skittles
9 Double-footed jumps over three hurdles of appropriate height
10 Jump to touch a basketball ring.

There are, of course, anaerobic endurance sessions which can be pursued outside game situations. First, Fartlek runs can be 'weighted' by cutting down the jog-rests between sprints and fast strides. Then there are sessions such as 60m × 10 'turn-arounds', when the player strides 60m, immediately turns around and strides back. Similarly, an 800m run consisting of 30m of strides and 30m of jogs all the way produces a similar effect. Another such session, a game-simulation, involves 60m × 10 strides, with 10 press-ups at the end of each run. All of these sessions aim to produce an anaerobic endurance effect. All are based on a sound platform of endurance fitness.

Match-fitness is not a purely physiological phenomenon. As we have said in the opening chapter, there is the essential element of muscle hardness, one which it is impossible to measure, but which is essential for match-fitness. During August most clubs increase the level of body contact in their practices and before the season starts there are invariably trials and practice matches, both of which develop this element of body hardness.

The season itself brings a weekly match and this brings with it a modification of training. The first is the Sunday recovery run/swim. This is a useful element in the development not so much of endurance fitness but of recovery from post-match fatigue. This should be a 'talking pace' run over 3 to 5 km, one which may have a modest aerobic effect but which is essentially aimed at post-match recovery.

As we have mentioned swimming, this is perhaps the appropriate time also to mention 'cross-training'. This means endurance training which does not involve running, training which is particularly valuable if running is impossible because of injury or bad weather. It is also of particular value to heavy players who may find Achilles tendon problems or calf-cramps during long runs. 'Cross-training' can mean swimming, cycling or rowing-ergometer work, exercise for the cardio-respiratory system without the problems of weight-bearing. The England team has found particular value in the computerised rowing ergometer which provides clear objective results and has the added value of upper body development. 'Cross-training' is particularly good in the maintenance (as distinct from the development) of endurance, which must be primarily running-based.

We would expect endurance fitness to develop, to be maintained and to be marginally increased throughout the season, with recovery monitored using the multi-stage shuttle-run test. Endurance training provides the central pillar upon which skill ultimately rests, and is the core of rugby training.

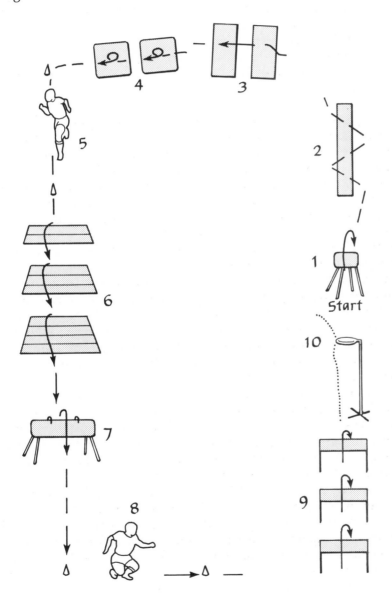

Table 8 Continuous Rugby Activity Circuit

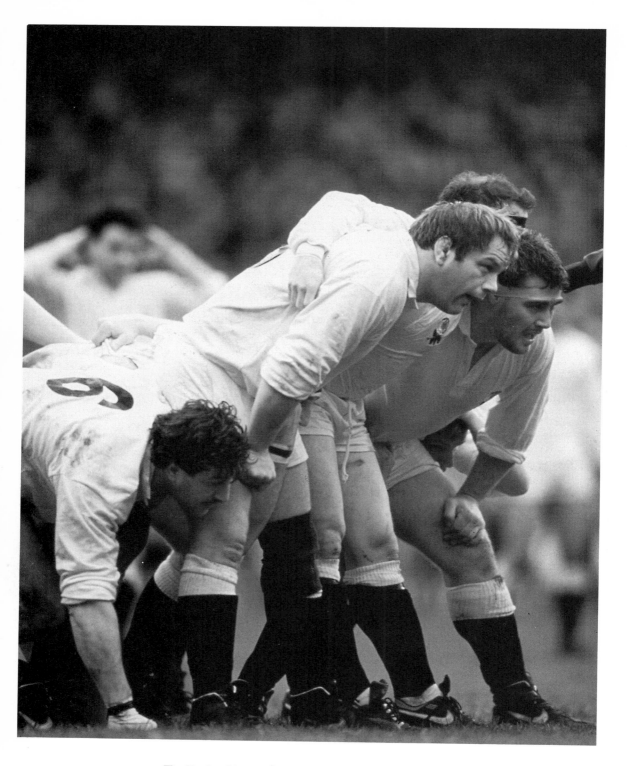

The England front row of Jeff Probyn, Brian Moore and Jason Leonard,
supported by flanker Mike Teague, prepares to pack down for a scrum.

Chapter 4

Strength

'Only the mediocre are always at their best'
(Jean Giradoux)

Strictly, strength is the ability to apply force against resistance, and involves no speed of contraction. However, in most sports this purely static activity rarely occurs on its own, in the sense that there is usually a speed of contraction element involved in every movement. A good example is a long-jump take-off where static strength is required at take-off to absorb the speed of the approach, then explosive strength to drive up and into the jump.

We can see that static strength (also called 'isometric strength') is particularly valuable to forwards who spend much time in static and semi-static scrummaging and mauling situations, but is of less value to backs.

Explosive power is clearly of particular value to backs, half-backs and back-row forwards, though clearly jumping power is vital to locks. When we move on to strength endurance (which is the ability of specific muscle groups to sustain repetitive activity), we can see that this is a priority for forwards rather than backs, simply because of the mauling/ripping demands of their position.

Again, as we have said in earlier chapters, everything comes back to the demands of the game. As an example, an international sprinter would undoubtedly have the accelerative power, as with a loose forward, to come off the back of scrums at pace, but he would be as limp as a lettuce after a bout of mauling, because of lack of contact fitness and of strength endurance in the trunk and arms. Similarly, an Olympic weight-lifter might produce great scrummaging thrust, but would not possess either the contact fitness or the levels of general endurance required to last out the 80 minutes of a match.

Strength training, like all other aspects of fitness training, is simply a process of muscular adaptation to the stress of working against resistance. Like all other forms of training, it will only produce good results if:

1 The techniques used are correct
2 The rest between exercises is adequate
3 Adequate rest between sessions is secured
4 The appropriate exercises are used, with the correct level of resistance
5 A good basic level of strength is achieved before specialised programmes are undertaken.

Strength training has much in common with sprint training, in that explosive power is required, and this means relatively small numbers of high-quality repetitions, at near-maximum effort, thus recruiting large numbers of muscle fibres. The level of intensity is based on what can be lifted in a single effort. For example, if we take a power clean, where a player can lift 100kg in a single lift, we may be looking at three sets of 8 × 80kg, with 2 minutes rest between sets. On re-testing, after 2 to 3 weeks, we find that the maximum has gone up to 110kg, and the weight lifted in sets then moves up to 85kg. If we take another example, a session on bench press, where the maximum lift is 110kg, we may be seeing a programme of 4 sets of 20 × 60kg, with 4 minutes rest between sets.

Table 9 sets out the various types of strength-training methods which now exist. These are a far cry from the rusting jumble of bar-bells and dumb-bells of recent memory. Many rugby clubs are now equipping themselves with the most sophisticated equipment available and most players can now gain access to commercial fitness centres containing apparatus capable of hitting every possible muscle group.

Table 9 Strength-training methods

1 Individual body resistance exercises
2 Body resistance exercises using equipment
3 Partner resistance exercises
4 Medicine balls (lifts, throws)
5 Circuit training
6 Plyometrics
7 Pulleys, springs and elastic bands
8 Free weights
9 Exercise machines
10 Isokinetic training
11 Isometric training

But the problem for the player, with possibly less than four hours per week of training time outside club sessions, is that of balancing out the needs of endurance, strength and speed in a manner compatible with leading a normal working and social life. To this end, simple circuits or limited weights sessions performed at the end of a club session, or even 'bread and butter' push-ups and abdominal exercises undertaken at home, may be the best that a player may be able to achieve.

It should be appreciated that in strength training the most available form of resistance is the body itself. There are a range of exercises which can be done individually or with a partner as body resistance exercises, and these can form a varied and demanding form of strength training. As no equipment is needed, they can be done easily on or beside the pitch with a group of players either before or after some other form of rugby training.

Body resistance exercises

This form of strength training simply involves altering the body position in order to vary the resistance against which a muscle or group of muscles is contracting. There are an unlimited number of exercises which can be used for upper body, abdominals and legs. The following section shows how resistance can be altered by a change of body position or with a partner to provide variety in one exercise – the push-up.

This was chosen as the example because of the need to develop upper body strength for the game of rugby football but the same approach can be adopted for any similar exercise. Examination of these exercises will show that resistances vary from an easy load in the kneeling push-up to a considerably increased load in the push-up from handstand using a partner. Also, some of the exercises, such as the clap-hand push-up, require movements which help to develop power.

Even though these are all simple exercises needing no equipment, a great range of strength work can be conducted for different parts of the body and different arrangements of sets and repetitions can be built into this form of strength training.

Push-up theme

1 *Kneeling push-up*: front support position, with arms shoulder-width apart; kneel with the knees immediately below the hips and the feet on the floor. Bend the arms to 'lower' the chest to the floor and return to the front support position (Fig 19)

2 *Extended kneeling push-up*: the same as Fig 19 but kneel with the knees positioned back from the hips, the feet raised and the lower legs crossed; bend the arms to lower the chest to the floor and return to the front support position

3 *Push-up*: front support with back straight (Fig 20)

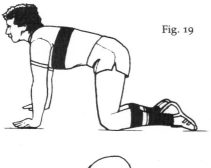

Fig. 19

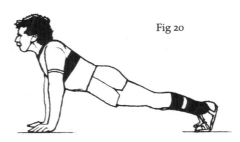

Fig 20

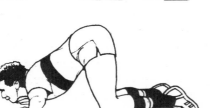

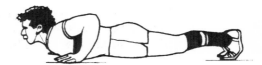

4 *Fingertip push-up*: the same as Fig 20 but with the weight on the fingertips

5 *Clap-hand push-up*: front support with back straight; push upwards quickly and clap hands in between push-ups (Fig 21)

6 *Push-up slapping chest*: the same as Fig 21 but push upwards quickly and touch the chest in between push-ups

7 *Push-up raising one leg*: front support with back straight; raise one leg each time the chest is lowered to the ground (Fig 22)

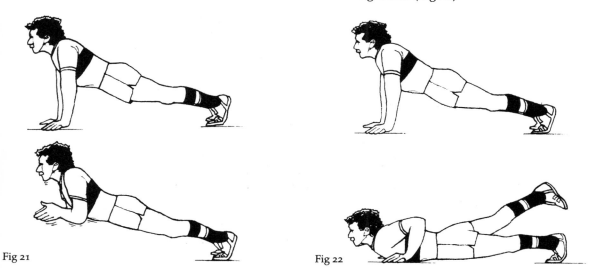

Fig 21

Fig 22

8 *One arm push-up*: front support with one hand behind the back (Fig 23)

9 *Extension push-up*: front support position with arms and legs extended (Fig 24)

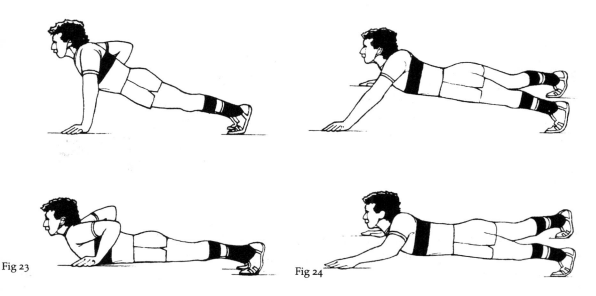

Fig 23

Fig 24

10 *Dips*: knees bent, feet flat on the ground, seat just above the floor, arms straight, palms on the floor and fingers pointing forward; bend the arms as much as possible until your seat touches the floor, then straighten your arms to return back to starting position (Fig 25)

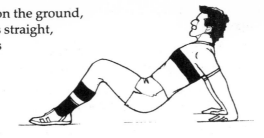

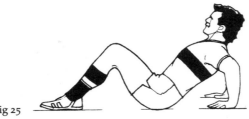

Fig 25

11 *Extended dips*: the same as Fig 25 but heels on the floor, legs, body and arms straight and fingers pointing forwards; bend arms as much as possible keeping your body straight, then straighten your arms to return to the starting position

12 *Push-up feet raised*: partner holds player's feet by his hips; player presses from full extensions of arms to touch the floor with his chest (Fig 26)

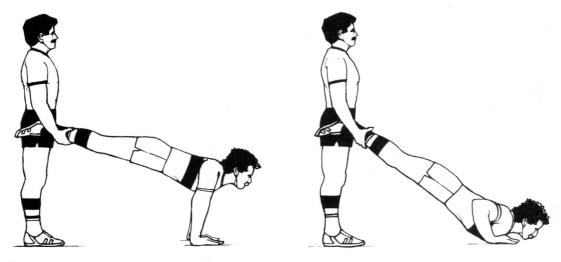

Fig 26

13 *Push-up feet raised higher*: the same as Fig 26 but partner holds player's feet on his shoulders; player presses from full extension of the arms to touch the floor with his chest.

49

14 *Combined push-up*: partner places his feet on player's shoulders with both in front support position; player presses from full extension of the arms to touch the floor with his chest (Fig 27)

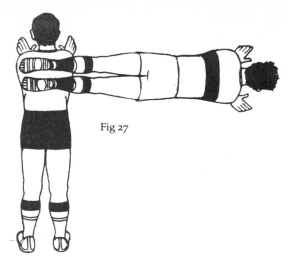

Fig 27

15 *Separate wrists*: player faces partner and holds his wrists with arms up in front of chest; player tries to pull wrists apart to the side (Fig 28)

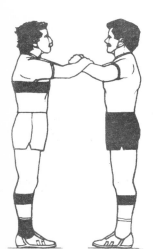

Fig 28

16 *Press hands*: player faces partner who holds arms out straight and to the side; player places hands outside partner's wrists and slowly forces the hands together (Fig 29a)

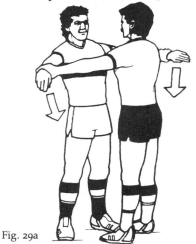

Fig. 29a

17 *Clap hands*: both players lie on their back, heads together and arms apart; partner has palms facing down, gripping player's wrists, and player has palms facing upwards; player slowly tries to raise his arms and clap his hands above his head (Fig 29b)

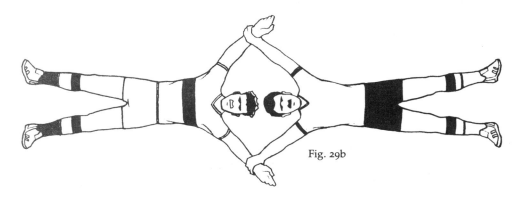

Fig. 29b

18 *Arm press and abdominal curl*: a player sits on his partner's shoulders with his feet tucked in between his partner's legs; the player leans back slowly to the horizontal as an extension trunk curl, then returns to sitting upright; this movement gradually places a resistance on the player's arms and shoulders (Fig 30).

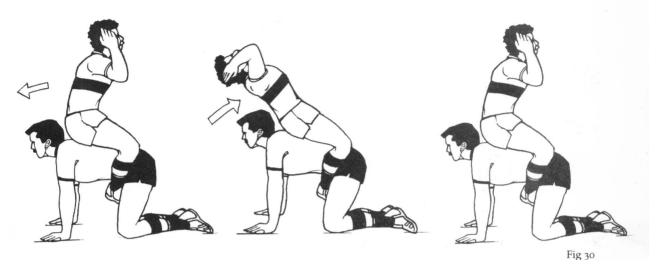

Fig 30

Static strength

As we said earlier, this rarely exists in a 'pure' form in any sport. If we look at Figs 32 and 33, showing a squat in weight-lifting, we can see that the muscles of the back work statically to hold the spine in the correct flat position. At this point in the lift, the muscles of the front of the thighs also work statically to fix the weight at right angles. When, however, the weight is driven vertically, the muscles of the thighs now work explosively, with those of the back still operating statically to fix the position. In some ways, this is similar to a scrummage where there is a static element at put-in, then an explosive horizontal drive with the legs, again operating through a flat back.

Static strength is best achieved by lifts in the 1 to 6 repetition area and overlaps with explosive strength at the 4 to 6 repetition level. Similarly, the exercises recommended in the next section, which relate to explosive strength, will in the same way overlap downwards into the static strength area. Thus, we recommended that props and locks (who have particular need for static strength) should move up into the 6+ repetition area as the static element will then be adequately catered for.

Explosive power

Explosive power is the combination of static (isometric) strength and speed of contraction. As we have previously said, static strength is rarely expressed on its own, being usually accompanied by an explosive

51

shortening of muscle fibres. Explosive power, therefore, is the most important means by which strength is expressed in rugby and appears in line-out jumping, for example, runs from standing starts, drives through tackles and loose and tight forward drives.

Weight training

There are a number of priority areas for strength training in rugby, such as the development of leg power, but we would suggest the following as core exercises. They are listed by areas of the body but some exercises work muscle groups in more than one area:

Legs	1 Power clean
	2 Back squat
	3 Front squat
	4 Hamstring curl
	5 High pull
Chest	6 Bench press
Back	7 Lat pull
Shoulders	8 Lateral dumb-bell raise
	9 Overhead military press
	10 Press behind neck
Arms	11 Bicep curl
	12 Tricep extension
Abdominals	13 Bent-leg sit-up with crossover

Power clean (Figs 31a, 31b, 31c)

Starting position: Adopt the basic standing start position for most weight-training exercises. The feet are slightly wider than hip-width apart, the heels flat on the floor and the toes turned slightly outwards. Place the insteps under the bar. Stand erect with the arms by your sides. Bend from the hips and knees to take up a crouch position and grip the bar using an overgrasp grip just wider than shoulder-width apart. Arms should remain straight and relaxed. Look up with the back flat and the seat as high as the position comfortably permits.

Action

1 Raise the bar by extending the legs and keeping the arms fully straight. Keep the bar close to the legs and press the thighs forward as the bar passes the knees. Keep the bar moving continuously close to the body, and when the bar reaches chest height drop the hips while bending at the knees, so lowering the shoulder to bar level.

2 Hands and forearms rotate under the bar to place it across the front of the chest with the palms upwards in the receiving position. Force

the elbows forward to rest the bar on the chest so as to avoid supporting the weight of the bar with the arms.

3 To return the bar to the floor, lower to the thighs and then to the floor.

4 Breathe in during the lift and breathe out as the bar is lowered.

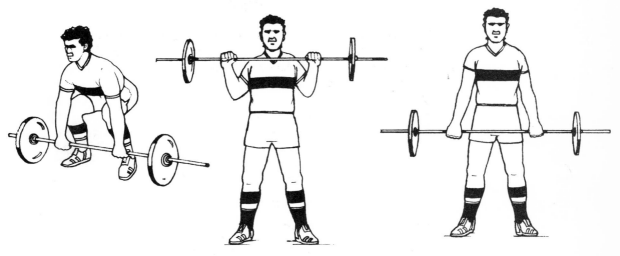

Fig 31a   Fig 31b   Fig 31c

Starting position: Adopt the shoulder rest starting position. The feet are slightly wider than hip-width apart and the bar is behind the neck, resting across the shoulders and the back of the neck. The head is up and the shoulders are braced back. Use an overgrasp grip with the hands more than shoulder-width apart and the elbows flexed.

Back squat (Figs 32a, 32b)

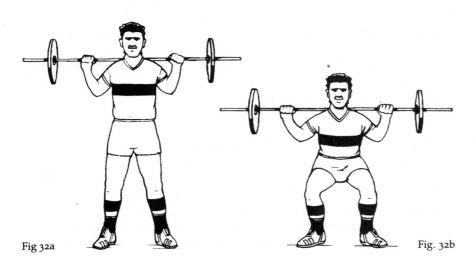

Fig 32a   Fig. 32b   **53**

Action

1 Maintaining a flat, upright back, lower the hips and bar by bending the legs while pushing the knees outwards. Keep the back as flat as possible and keep the head pressed back. Control the downward movement until the thighs are parallel to the floor. It is inadvisable to lower further.

2 Powerfully lift the weight back to the starting position. Straighten the legs and press the hips forward under the bar in order to maintain a strong lifting position.

3 Breathe in on lowering and breathe out on lifting.

4 Try to keep the feet flat on the floor throughout the movement. If this is difficult in the low position due to a lack of flexibility in the ankle flexors, place a disc weight or 3cm-thick block of wood under both heels at the start.

5 Spotters are advised, particularly when using heavier weights, to assist with taking the bar-bell on to the shoulders and to help in controlling the weight if required. In some facilities, safety racks or squat stands are included to help with this type of exercise.

Front squat (Fig 33)

Starting position: As for the back squat but the bar is now resting across the front of the shoulders and the top of the chest, with the elbows held high and hands slightly wider than shoulder-width apart.

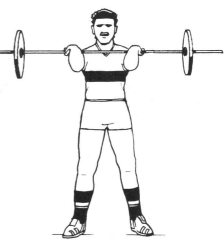

Action: Same as for the back squat. This exercise develops leg, hip and back strength and it places greater demands on the quadriceps than the back squat. It exercises the main muscle groups: quadriceps, gluteus maximus, erector spinae, biceps brachii.

Fig 33

Hamstring curl (Fig 34)

Starting position: Lie face down on the bench with the backs of the ankles under the higher padded roll. Grip the bars with both hands. The head should be raised comfortably and the spine as flat as possible.

Action

1 Lift the heels and pull the bar towards the buttocks as far as possible.

2 Slowly lower the weight back down to the starting position, where the hamstrings are comfortably stretched.

3 Breathe in as the knees flex and breathe out as they extend to lower the weight down.

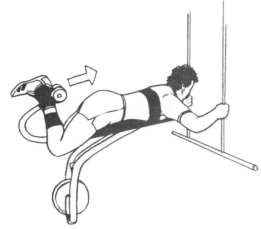

Fig 34

Starting position: As for the clean.

High pull (Figs 35a, 35b)

Action

   1 Raise the bar by extending the legs powerfully, then rise on the toes as the bar is pulled to the chin in one continuous movement.
   2 In the upper position the legs should be fully extended with the heels raised. The arms are out to the side, with the elbows flexed and the wrists above the bar also flexed.
   3 Return the bar to the floor carefully and under control.
   4 Breathe in during the lift and out as the bar is lowered.

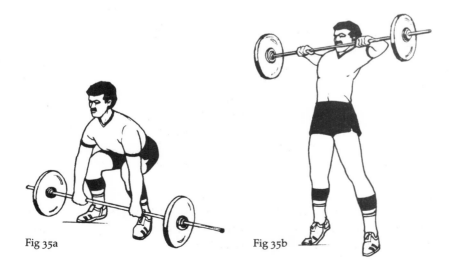

Fig 35a   Fig 35b

55

Bench press (Figs 36a, 36b, 36c)

Starting position: Adopt the supine starting position. Lie on the bench with the knees bent at right angles and the feet resting firmly on the ground and turned slightly outwards. The hips, shoulders and head should be kept on the bench throughout the exercise.

Action

1 The bench press is an exercise which requires the use of support racks or two spotters, with clear communication as to when the bar is to be exchanged between the player and the spotters at the beginning and end of the exercise.

2 Before taking the bar from the racks or spotters, the hands, using overgrasp, should be positioned on the bar so that it is well balanced and the arms are outstretched.

3 With the palms under and supporting the bar, take the weight and lower under control to the chest, then press upwards to straighten the arms fully.

4 Breathe in when lowering the bar and breathe out as the arms straighten.

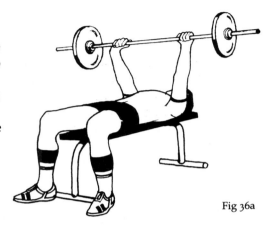

Fig 36a

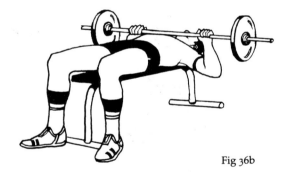

Fig 36b

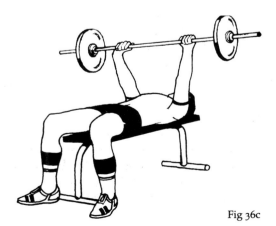

Fig 36c

Starting position: Sit securely on the seat, allowing the spine to stretch fully with the bar above the head. Use the wide overgrasp grip on the bar

Lat pull (Fig 37)

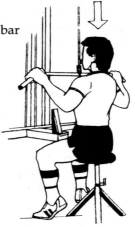

Action

1 Slowly pull the bar down in front of the face. Draw elbows downwards to the sides and bring the bar just below the chin.
2 Allow the weight to return by slowly letting the bar rise back to the start position.
3 Breathe in as you pull down and breathe out as the weight is controlled back.

Fig 37

Starting position: Stand with the feet slightly more than hip-width apart. Hold a dumb-bell in each hand with the palms facing inwards.

Lateral dumb-bell raise (Figs 38a, 38b)

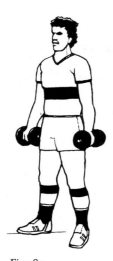
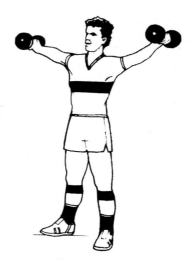

Fig 38a   Fig 38b

Action

1 Keeping the arms straight, raise the dumb-bells sideways to a position where the weights are slightly higher than shoulder level. Do not swing the weight, use the shoulders.
2 Lower the dumb-bells back to the sides.
3 Breathe in as the dumb-bells are raised and breathe out as they are lowered.

57

Overhead military press (Fig 39a, 39b)

Starting position: Clean the bar to the 'chest rest position', that is, the end position of the 'clean', previously described. The bar rests on the upper chest with an overgrasp grip slightly more than shoulder-width apart and with the hands under the bar. The elbows are flexed and pointing forward; the legs and back are straight with the feet placed comfortably slightly wider than hip-width apart.

Action

1 Press the bar to full arm extension directly above the head. Keep the legs and back straight throughout. Balance and control are essential for this movement as the weight is carried high above the head.
2 Lower the bar slowly back to the chest rest position.
3 Breathe in on pressing the bar and breathe out on lowering the bar.

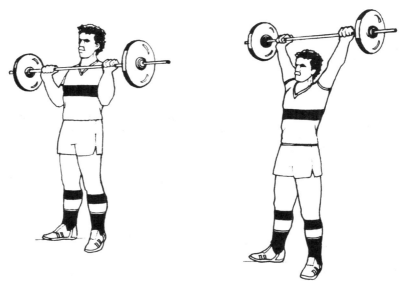

Fig 39a   Fig 39b

Press behind neck (Fig 40)

Starting position: As for the military press but hold the bar across the back of the neck and shoulders.

Action

1 Press upwards to a full arm extension directly above the head. As with the military press, maintain good balance and control, keeping the legs and back straight.

2 Lower the bar slowly and carefully back to rest on the back of the neck and shoulders.

3 Breathe in on pressing the bar and breathe out on lowering the bar.

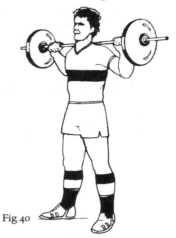

Fig 40

Starting position: Adopt the thigh support position using an undergrasp grip with the hands about shoulder-width apart. Keep the legs and back straight with the shoulders pulled back.

Bicep curl
(Figs 41a, 41b)

Action

1 Raise the bar by slowly flexing the arms until the bar reaches the chest, keeping the elbows still and against the sides of the trunk. Keep the head up throughout the exercise.

2 Lower the bar slowly back to the starting position.

3 Breathe in when lifting the bar and breathe out when lowering the bar.

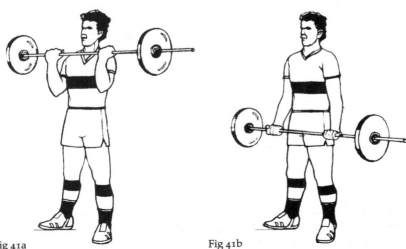

Fig 41a   Fig 41b

59

Tricep extension
(Fig 42)

Starting position: Take hold of the bar using an overgrasp grip. The stance should be comfortable with the back straight.

Action
1 Push the bar down to arm's length with the elbows tucked close into the sides of the body.
2 Control the bar back to the starting position.
3 Breathe in as the bar is pushed down and breathe out as it is brought back to the starting position.

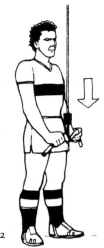

Fig 42

Bent-leg sit-up with crossover
(Fig 43)

These should be performed with knees bent (at 90 degrees) and feet flat on the floor and unanchored. The hands can be placed either on the shoulders with arms folded across the body, or next to the ears with elbows pointed forwards. Curl up to place the right elbow on the left knee and/or, on the next repetition, the left elbow on the right knee.

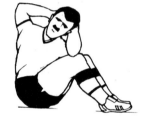

Fig 43

Repetitions

Try to do 6 to 10 repetitions in each set. You will need to work with a load which you can just manage to lift the required number of times (the last 3 should be tough). With abdominal work try to do a certain amount of repetitions, say 20 to 30, in each of 3 sets.

Sets

Try eventually to complete 3 sets. Start with 2, then build up; rest for 2 to 3 minutes between each set.

Exercises

Do 6 to 10 different exercises at each session. You should stick to a regular programme of exercises but you can add other exercises for variety and to place an emphasis on a particular area, such as the arms, for example.

Progression

Try to increase the load you are lifting every 2 to 3 weeks. As a guide, if you are doing repetitions of 10 when you complete 13 repetitions on the final set of an exercise, then increase the load a little. In order to keep track of your progress, try to fill in a weight-training card during or soon after each session.

Name	Personal Weight	Position

PHASE OF TRAINING		

Duration of Training	From:	To:

Date					
Exercise			—	REPETITION MAXIMUM	
Sets					
Reps					
Kg					
Exercise			—	REPETITION MAXIMUM	
Sets					
Reps					
Kg					
Exercise			—	REPETITION MAXIMUM	
Sets					
Reps					
Kg					

Table 10 Weight Training Record Card

Order

You should exercise the larger muscle groups first, working towards smaller muscles later. You will generally do this if you exercise the areas of the body in this order:

Legs ● Chest ● Back ● Shoulders ● Arms ● Abdominals

Rest

It is advisable to leave at least 48 hours between strength sessions so that muscles can fully recover and become stronger following resistance training. You can do strength sessions on consecutive days provided you work different muscle groups in each session.

Plyometrics

Plyometrics have been used with success in track and field athletics over the past quarter of a century, particularly in the power events of throwing, jumping, hurdling and sprinting.

Many rugby players have undertaken a weight training programme and have, as a result, increased their maximum strength or static strength. They have not, however, necessarily developed the specific power which is required in so many situations in the game – jumping in the line-out, driving forward in the ruck or maul, sprinting from a standing start.

Plyometrics has been found to bridge the gap between sheer strength and the power needed to produce these explosive, powerful movements. Power is a factor of strength and speed. Strength is increased through resistance training, which increases the cross-sectional area of the muscle and enhances the recruitment and firing rates of its motor units. It is important that a player has a very good strength base before undertaking plyometric training. Speed is increased by repetitive activities which maximise contraction time (see Chapter 5). The theory behind plyometrics is that maximum tension develops when a muscle is stretched quickly. The faster a muscle is forced to lengthen, the greater the tension it exerts. The rate of stretch is more important than the magnitude of the stretch, but the more a muscle is pre-stretched before contraction occurs the greater force it can apply.

A sequence of plyometric exercises is demanding on the muscles and the joints because of the explosive nature of the work. As in weight training, it is essential that there is adequate warm-up and that the proper techniques are used. Each repetition of a plyometric movement must be performed with maximal effort; the force should be applied in a continuous and consistent manner, with the emphasis on the speed of the movement.

The essence of plyometrics is quick recoil. There is no point in dwelling on the ground on landing or in taking an extra recovery bounce because the value of the exercise is then lost.

Plyometrics should be done in sets, in the same way as sprint drills, with 2 to 3 minutes rest between sets. The number of repetitions for each exercise can vary from 6 to 10 and the number of sets may vary between 3 and 6. Because of the stress on muscles, ligaments and tendons, sufficient periods of rest should be planned between sessions. A cool-down is always necessary to assist the recovery process after training. As a guide, 2 or possibly 3 sessions per week would seem to give the best results.

We would recommend that surfaces should be flat, firm and resilient. This means firm grass and, when gymnasiums are used, the use of mats for landings.

The following plyometric exercises are for the legs and upper body, though emphasis should be placed mainly on leg work:

With feet placed about shoulder-width apart and
hands down by the sides, begin the movement
by quickly lowering to a half-squat position,
then check this downward movement by
exploding upwards as high as possible
and throwing the arms upwards to
assist the take-off. Upon landing
repeat the movement and work
for maximum height each time.

Squat jump
(Fig 44)

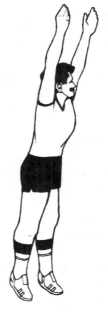

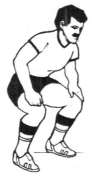

Fig 44

Drop to a quarter-squat and immediately explode upwards, trying to
touch the palms of the hands with the knees. On touching the ground,
treat it as if it was a red-hot stove and drive upwards.

Knee tucks
(Fig 45)

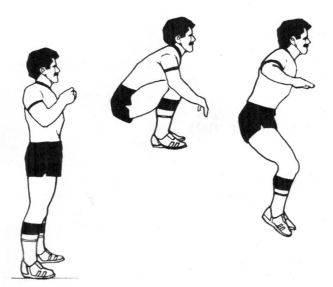

Fig 45

Split jumps
(Fig 46)

Adopt a starting position, one leg extended, forward leg flexed to 90 degrees. Spring up and, on regaining position, spring up again. An alternative is scissor-jumps, where there is an alternate leg-split.

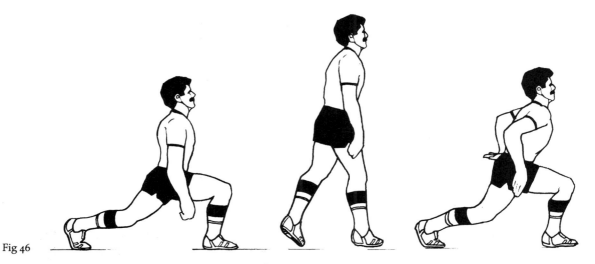

Fig 46

Multiple jumps
(Fig 47)

Jog in slowly, the trunk vertical, then make flat-footed bounds, maintaining posture, stressing high knee-swing and a feel of cling, cling, cling, with the grounded foot. Do this over a distance of 20 to 50m.

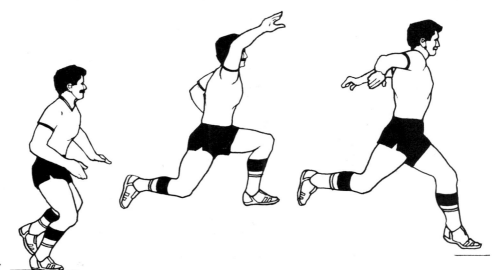

64   Fig 47

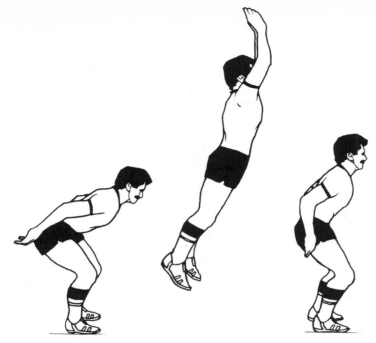

Fig 48

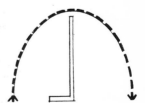

Stand with the feet comfortably apart and knees bent in the half-squat position, arms at the side and shoulders forward over the knees. Jump forward and upwards, driving from the hips and knees while swinging the arms forward. Try to get as much height and distance as possible and straighten the body in the air. Upon landing bend the knees and repeat the movement.

Double-leg bound (Fig 48)

This exercise requires a set of hurdles of appropriate height about 1m apart. Face the first hurdle with the feet comfortably apart. Begin by lowering the body, then jump explosively with both feet together and keeping the knees high over the first hurdle. On landing, continue the movements over the remaining hurdles, concentrating on driving the knees upwards and swinging the arms forwards.

Double-leg hurdle jump (Fig 49)

Fig 49

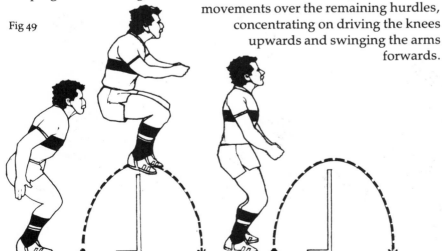

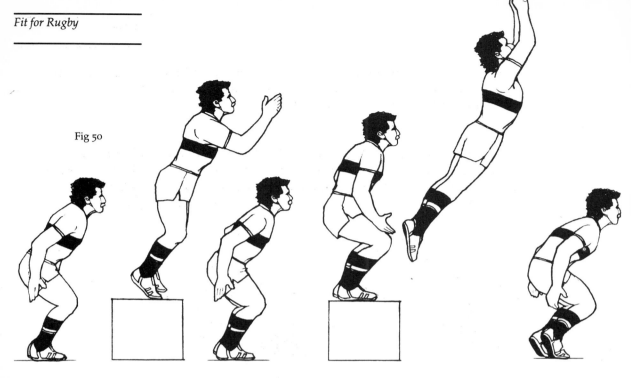

Box bounds
(Fig 50)

This calls for four boxes, 40 to 70cm high, placed 1 to 1.5m apart, and a soft landing surface. Jump up on the box and spring high from it, with full extension. On landing, recoil immediately and explosively, up on to the next box.

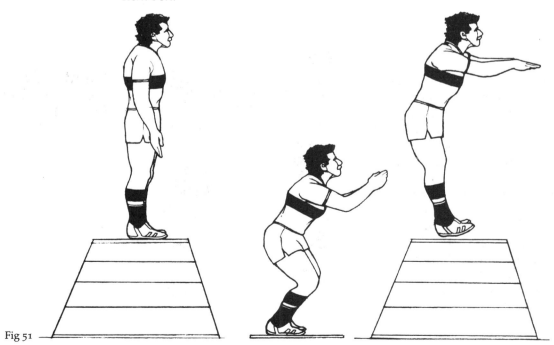

Depth jump
(Fig 51)

Set out two boxes at a suitable height with a mat in between. Drop from one box to land with both feet together. On contact with the floor bend the knees and jump explosively up on to the next vaulting box.

Dumb-bell alternate arm swing
(Fig 52)

Stand with the feet comfortably apart and the knees slightly bent, holding a dumb-bell of suitable weight in each hand. Swing the arm forwards and upwards to above the shoulder while taking the other arm backwards. Check the movement at the end of each swing and reverse the direction.

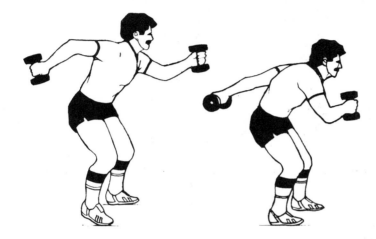

Fig 52

Dumb-bell vertical swing
(Fig 53)

Stand with the feet shoulder-width apart, knees bent, and hold a dumb-bell of suitable weight (or other suitable object) in both hands between the legs. Keep the back straight and the head up. Swing the dumb-bell upwards. Keeping the arms straight and letting the body extend. At the top of the swing quickly change direction and pull the dumb-bell down. Keep repeating these movements continuously.

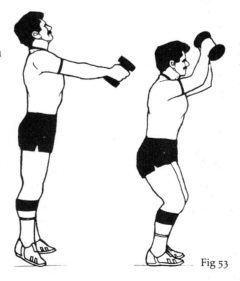

Fig 53

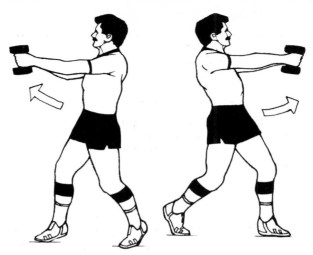

Fig 54

Dumb-bell horizontal swing (Fig 54)

Stand with the feet shoulder-width apart and the arms extended out in front of the chest, holding a dumb-bell of suitable weight in both hands. Pull the dumb-bell to one side and allow the trunk to twist. At the end of the swing quickly check the movement and pull the dumb-bell in the other direction. Continue these movements from side to side.

Table 11 Plyometrics – reminders

1 Landing – recoils must be fast!
2 Good technique must be observed
3 Adequate rests between sets must be observed
4 Work out in training shoes with strong foot support and use a good surface – grass or mats
5 End the session if the legs become fatigued
6 Begin a plyometric programme only when a good strength-base has been established

Table 12 The Ten Commandments of strength training

1 Never play around in a gym. Respect the equipment.
2 Allow two hours after a meal for a session, so that digestion is complete.
3 Make sure that collars are firm and pins correctly inserted in the holes of weight-stacks.
4 Build slowly in your programme, by starting in a general high-repetition schedule.
5 Establish breathing rhythms, always breathing out on the effort.
6 Work out at least twice a week for strength development, once for strength maintenance.
7 Never work out if you have any form of viral illness.
8 Maintain the warm-up, core exercises and cool-down ritual.
9 Always wear a lifting belt when using free weights.
10 Always work with partners when using free weights.

Chapter 5

Speed

'He's so fast he can put out the light
and get into bed before it's dark'
(Anon)

It is often thought that speed is a 'natural' quality, and one which is therefore resistant to improvement. In essence, you are either fast or you are not. There is some truth in this. We all know of young athletes capable of running around 11 seconds for 100m without having done anything much in the way of training. The equivalent performance in an endurance activity, an untrained run of 4 minutes 25 seconds for 1,500 metres, is much less common.

It is certainly true that speed is less susceptible to improvement than endurance. Our young 11-seconds 100m runner may improve, with hard training, to 10.20 to 10.40 seconds, an improvement of 6/8 per cent. In contrast, our 4 minutes 25 seconds, 1,500m runner may well improve with training to around 3 minutes 40 seconds, an improvement closer to 20 per cent. The endurance systems used by the middle distance athletes, which are much more comprehensive than the skeletal muscular system used by the sprinter, are consequently capable of much greater change. There is the added factor in endurance activities of the psychological element, the capacity to tolerate fatigue, one which is learned with training.

It is fair to say, therefore, that the 14-seconds 100m prop is never going to run even 12 seconds, whatever his training programme. Nevertheless, it is possible to improve speed substantially and this chapter is dedicated to that end.

Speed over 100m is not, in any case, the appropriate test for a rugby player. Instead we should be concerned with speed in the 15 to 50m area, those being distances which all studies show are the most frequently covered in the game.

Types of speed

There are three basic types of speed:
1 Accelerative speed (up to 30m)
2 Pure speed (60m)
3 Speed endurance (repeated sprints)

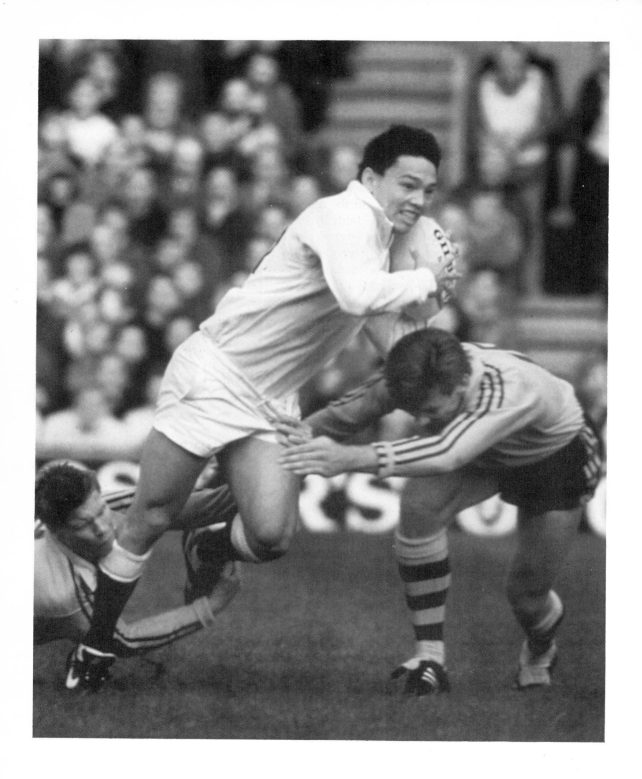

Rory Underwood uses his speed and strength to burst through
the tackles of Australia's Nick Farr-Jones and Andrew Leeds.

Of these, accelerative speed is very important for the rugby player. A scrum-half driving forward with the ball off the base of the scrum, a wing forward launching himself towards his opposing stand-off, a prop pumping forward with the ball, all these are examples of accelerative speed. It will be noted that two of them are ball-carrying examples, but we would observe that most rugby-running is done without the ball, in support situations, in covering or in making tackles.

One example of improvement in accelerative speed will show its value. Back in 1986 when Bath's Richard Hill first became England's scrum-half, his speeds over 30m were around 4.20 seconds, slower than at least one England lock, Steve Bainbridge, who ran the distance in 3.94 seconds. This lack of speed limited Richard's ability to make runs and as a consequence his game tended to centre around passing or working the ball back into his back row. Improvements in accelerative speed in 1987–88, however, brought him inside 4.00 seconds and his running game has brought a new and important dimension to his play by providing him with a greater number of options.

The testing schedule now practised by the England team and described in Chapter 9 uses 15m and 30m as the test-distances, and we have seen during the period between 1986 and 1991 significant improvements, particularly over the longer distances.

The fact that accelerative speed is a major factor in rugby does not, however, mean that all training takes place over 30m. This is for three reasons:

1 Some positions (centres, wings, full-backs) do make occasional runs over longer distances
2 In situations where the backs have to make successive runs, they may have 30m/45m/50m looped together in a short space of time, often with little rest; this means speed endurance
3 Much running in rugby, particularly by the forwards, is at cruising speed over 50m to 60m. The higher the basic speed, the higher the cruising speed.

Methods

Table 13 shows the methods which can be used to develop the various elements of speed. Some of these methods, such as weight training and plyometrics, are covered in other chapters and although we refer to them here, the diagrammatic detail of these exercises will be shown in the appropriate chapters.

It can be seen also from Table 13 that the development of speed is not simply a matter of marking out a 30m stretch and blasting out a succession of sprints. True, specific types of running will produce specific speed elements, but one type of speed practice invariably overlaps with another. So it must be remembered that although 30 metres is probably the distance most frequently sprinted in the game, this is not always done

71

from a standing start, but often from a jog or stride. And, of course, running distances longer than 30m will have some impact upon speed in the shorter 30m distance.

The 'direct' methods shown in Table 13 involve an immediate transfer to sprinting and are exclusive, while the 'indirect' methods (such as weight training and plyometrics) are methods which, though they will improve sprinting speed, also apply to almost every other aspect of training and will therefore come up again and again. Let us now look at each aspect in more detail.

Table 13

Element	Direct training	Indirect training
Accelerative speed	1 Uphill sprints (30–50m) 2 Sprints from standing start (20–30m) 3 Speed drills from standing start (30m)	Plyometrics Weight training (6 to 10 repetitions)
Pure speed	1 Speed drills (40–60m) 2 90%–100% effort runs over 50–60m in sets of 4 to 6	Plyometrics Weight training (10 to 15 repetitions)
Speed endurance	1 Speed drills (60–80m) 2 90%–100% effort runs over 60–100m in sets of 3 to 6	Plyometrics Weight training (sets of 10 to 15 repetitions) Circuit training
Change of pace	1 Acceleration runs at 90%–100% 2 Speed drills 3 'Hollow' sprints 4 Effort-level runs	

Accelerative speed

Acceleration is the period when the body is being moved from inertia; it is therefore a high impulse/high ground contact period. This means that it differs from pure sprinting, where the player is already moving and the contact time is therefore much lower. Thus, hill-running on modest inclines which increases contact time and which encourages vigorous leg-extensions is included in the 'direct' session. Hill-running also encourages the strong use of the arms and this is an aspect which will be fully dealt with later in the 'speed drills' section.

A sprint from a standing start is an activity which explains itself. One of our basic tenets is that muscles 'learn' speed and that one of the best ways for this learning to be achieved is simply to perform short-distance starts. If we can add to that the skill element involved, using elements of the 'speed drills', then the learning process is complete.

All sprinting is a high-quality activity and the focus of attention must therefore be high and the rests between sets relatively long. We are therefore looking at sets of between 4 and 6 in the 30m to 60m sprints, with rests of at least 5 minutes between sets. When fatigue sets in, quality drops and there is a danger of injury.

When distances are above 60m (for example, in the speed endurance section), then rests between runs must naturally be longer (3 to 5 minutes) and rests between sets longer (7 minutes or more). Again, the aim is to keep up the quality of the work, otherwise the objective is lost, and the session begins to become interval training.

It is essential, too, to perform all sprinting on good-quality surfaces, such as flat grass, cinder or a synthetic track. If a grass training surface is soft and wet, the practice must take place in boots; if it is dry, then road-shoes with a good grip will be fine.

Pure speed

Here, as in all other speed practices, the effort level must be at 80 per cent or above. Once the period of basic conditioning has been achieved, the emphasis should always be on operating at close to full speed. This means that the volume must inevitably be low, not more than 1,200m per session. It involves, for example, a series of repetition sprints, such as 3 sets of 60m × 6 with slow walk-back recovery, 5 minutes rest between sets, or 4 sets of 40m × 5 with the same rest periods. As in all other speed sessions, the level of attention must be high and working with other players of the same ability will help to keep the quality at the right level.

Speed endurance

In the first chapter we made it clear that most full-speed running in rugby rarely goes beyond 30m. There are, however, occasional longer runs, particularly by wingers and full-backs. There are occasional high-speed activity chains, for example, 30m/20m/30m, which make demands on speed endurance. Thus, sessions going beyond 60m are of value, though even 'pure' speed sessions, such as 3 sets of 60m × 6, do have a speed endurance effect, and an effect on accelerative speed.

Change of pace

If anything differentiates rugby-running from that of athletics it is change of pace. Athletic sprinting is essentially one pace, which is eyeballs-out. However, such factors as the element of deception in running at an opponent or coming into the line at high speed means that rugby-running is often made at varying speeds. One practice for this is 'hollow sprinting' which uses two sprints interrupted by a period of recovery in the form of light running or jogging. You may accelerate 20 to 30m, then accelerate again up to full pace, then walk for 100 to 150m as the recovery phase. Sets of this sequence can then be adopted.

This form of sprint training is appropriate to rugby players with its

73

variation in speed and tempo during one sequence and, though clearly aimed at change of pace, has an overlap effect upon pure speed and upon speed endurance.

A second practice consists of acceleration sprints or 'gear-change' running, which involve a gradual increase from a rolling start, to jogging, to striding out and to full pace; the rest interval should then be a walk-back recovery and 3 to 6 sprints per set and 2 or more sets per session can be used. This method is very useful for emphasising and maintaining the technical component of the sprinting action as the pace increases. Players can use the try line, 22-metre line and the half-way line as markers for increase in speed. Again this form of sprint training has implications for 'pure' speed and speed endurance.

Acceleration running is a further modification to the training, involving a gradual increase in speed over a given distance always beyond 60 metres. The feeling is of a gradual increase in effort and the practice therefore differs from the sudden 'gear changes' of the previous method.

Speed drills

Speed drills are at the very heart of the speed programme. In essence, they take out each part of the sprint action, refine it, control it and focus it. By this means we can make even the most stolid prop if not into a racehorse, then certainly into a speedier carthorse. Let's look at speed drills in detail.

First, they take place over a distance of 40 to 60m, giving us an extra speed and speed endurance pay-off. This distance should be on a running track or flat grass and the 'running territory' should be clearly marked out with cones so that the focus is intense. Finally, all effort should be in the region of 80 to 100 per cent. In early season training they should tend towards 80 per cent and, as the muscles become conditioned, they can then move closer to 100 per cent. The principal aim of the drills is to achieve efficient movement of arms and legs about a still head and trunk.

1 *Hip and shoulder fix*: Here the player jogs in on the starting line, hips high, on the balls of his feet. The feeling is of flat, low shoulders. So the 'feel' is high hips, low shoulders (Fig 55).

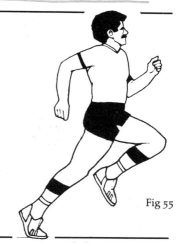

Fig 55

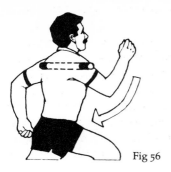

2 *Arm positioning*: The 'feel' here is of a steel pin through the shoulders (Fig 56). The feeling is of the arms rotating loosely around this steel pin, 'lip to hip'. This means that the hand rises to lip level and comes back just beyond the hip. This, in effect, accurately positions the hands and dictates the range of the arms.

Fig 56

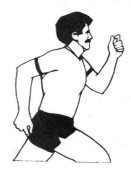

Fig 57

3 *'Potato crisp' hands*: Now we move to more detail. The focus is now on the hands, with the feeling being one of holding a potato crisp between thumb and index finger (Fig 57). The crisp must *not* be broken, so there must be relaxation of hand and wrist. This is a simple practice, but it often has dramatic effects because of the relaxation which it produces.

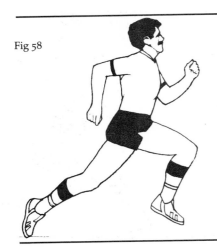

Fig 58

4 *Elbow drive*: Here the emphasis is on the vigorous driving back of the elbows (Fig 58). An extension of this drill is the 'acceleration run on arms' drill. Here the emphasis is on gradually increasing the elbow drive throughout the length of the run.

5 *Jelly jaw*: Watch a great sprinter, at the height of his powers, running in slow motion. You will see little sign of effort, for the muscles of the face and neck are loose and relaxed. Here, in this practice, we try to secure maximum relaxation or 'jelly jaw' (Fig 59). The feeling is of a jaw which hangs loose, of a wobbly lip. This is a practice which can be run at 80 per cent, then put under pressure at full effort when the player feels that he has achieved the necessary relaxation control at lower speeds.

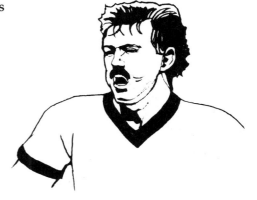

Fig 59

6 *Driving practice*: This is a drill which must be practised on a firm surface. It is essentially an acceleration drill and should be worked on over 30m. From a standing start, both toes pointing forward, the player drives out, trying to maintain contact with the ground as long as possible on each stride (Fig 60). The feeling is of 'cling, cling, cling'. The elements of elbow drive and 'jelly jaw' can be fed in as other focus points on this practice as it develops.

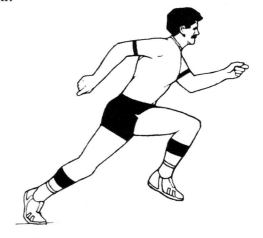

Fig 60

7 *Leg speed drill*: Marginal changes in leg speed can be important in rugby, in such situations as taking a pass coming into the line or in changing direction. The first practice simply involves running flat out, stressing cadence rather than range. To enable differentiation between range and cadence, we have a second practice. This involves running on full range for 20 to 30m, then turning on leg speed for the next 20 to 30m. It must be remembered that increased leg speed does *not* mean running on the spot, rather a marginal quickening of cadence (Fig 61).

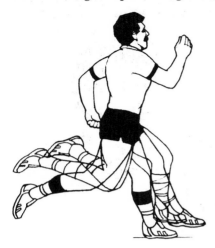

Fig 61

8) *High knee practice*: Here the player jogs in, knees high, then picks up speed, trying to keep the same high knee lift. An alternative practice is to stride 20 to 30m at 80 per cent effort, then 'lift' into a high knee action at full speed over the final 20 to 30m (Fig 62).

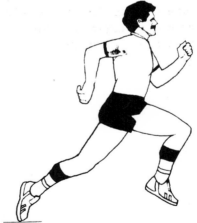

Fig 62

It can be seen that speed is almost infinite in its variety of activity, with at the centre the speed drills which produce a stable, relaxed running technique. No one can transform himself from a carthorse into a racehorse but anyone, repeat anyone, can substantially improve his running speed.

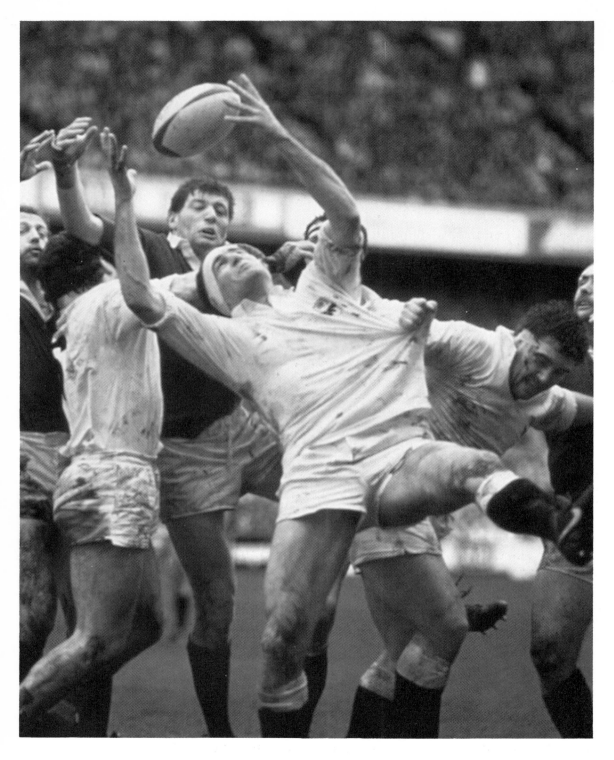

Paul Ackford demonstrates his flexibility in claiming
line-out ball against Ireland at Lansdowne Road in 1991.

Chapter 6

Flexibility

Although it is not always appreciated by the rugby player, there is considerable value in regular flexibility training. Flexibility has an influence on skilled movement because certain skills may be enhanced by an increase in range of movement.

Regular flexibility training can increase relaxation in the muscles and there is also some evidence to show that stretching exercises can help to ease the muscular soreness which follows a match or a hard training session.

Most players have experienced the frustration of missing games through injury and there is a wealth of data which confirms the value of flexibility training in preventing muscle and connective tissue injuries. So it is important that flexibility is developed to allow the optimum performance of certain skills in the game and as an effective means of injury-prevention.

There are basically two types of flexibility. First, 'static flexibility', which relates to the range of movement possible around a joint, and results from the stretching of muscles and connective tissue in that area. In contrast, 'dynamic flexibility' describes a player's ability to use a range of joint movement in the performance of a physical skill at various speeds.

To gain most benefit from flexibility work, it is helpful to understand the nature and structure of a flexibility training programme. First, a player needs to distinguish between a flexibility programme which will increase his range of movement in particular joints over a period of time; and one which is incorporated within warm-up and cool-down routines. The latter, performed immediately before and after training sessions or matches to prepare the body for activity, helps with the recovery process and reduces the risk of injury.

Flexibility training

Special stretching exercises and drills have been developed to increase the range of movement in various joints. These involve stretching the muscle beyond its habitual length. The two main methods of stretching exercises are categorised as 'ballistic' and 'static'.

Ballistic

Ballistic stretching involves a bobbing, bouncing and rhythmic movement, with momentum taking the moving limb or part of the body to its limits. Ballistic stretching can be used with the team during a stretching session or warm-up to work through a range of exercises together in a short period of time, promoting team togetherness. Ballistic stretching can also help to develop dynamic flexibility, and because most skills and movements are ballistic in nature, this type of fast stretching is helpful because of its specificity.

Although ballistic stretching can be less boring than static stretching, it is less likely to increase significantly the range of movement. This is because the quick, repetitive bouncing actions will initiate a stretch reflex, allowing only a momentary lengthening of the muscle. It is also possible for these exercises, if done incorrectly, to produce muscle-soreness and even losses in elasticity.

Static

Static stretching involves slow sustained exercises which place the muscle in a lengthened position under stretch and hold the position for a number of seconds. Static and slow stretching are preferable to ballistic stretching, as permanent lengthening of muscle is more likely following stretching of longer duration.

Static stretching is preferable also because it requires less energy expenditure and will probably result in less muscle-soreness. Although the argument supports static stretching, a good solution to the problem is to employ a sensible combination of both methods, with an awareness of the limitations and dangers of ballistic stretching.

The approach to flexibility training

1 Warm up well before you begin the routine of flexibility exercises, as muscles are more pliable and receptive to stretch if they are warm. It is also important to be fully relaxed during flexibility training and this is helped by an increase in body temperature. A suitable way to warm up is a period of light jogging followed by some light exercises. If training is taking place outside in cold conditions, then a track-suit should be worn, so that the increased body temperature can be maintained.

2 It is important to develop a sound technique for flexibility exercises. The aim is to ease gently into stretch position to a point where a comfortable tension is felt in the muscle. There is minimum strain, maximum relaxation, and no pain. When the muscles are being stretched, the feeling should be at worst one of 'mild discomfort' – nothing more.

3 The aim is to hold the stretch position for about 10 to 20 seconds and as the feeling of stretching decreases over that time stretch a little further but always remain comfortable. There is no bounce or jerk – only a steady, prolonged stretch.

4 As the player becomes more familiar with the technique of stretching, the aim should be to try to concentrate the point of stretch in the bulky central part of the muscle rather than near the joints where stress would be put on ligaments and tendons.

5 As it is important to stay relaxed during a flexibility routine, it helps if the player breathes calmly and rhythmically.

6 Regular flexibility work is recommended for a fitness training programme. The rate of improvement is largely influenced by the amount of flexibility work done, but 3 sessions per week would be a typical schedule. As it is a relatively easy form of training to do, requiring minimum facilities, one session per day is possible and should bring a marked improvement. The ideal time for some of the flexibility sessions would be after a training session when the body and muscles are warmed up from the previous work-out.

Static stretching exercises

The exercises can be done actively or passively. Active stretching involves working alone on flexibility exercises. In any movement or exercise one muscle acts as a prime mover, causing the movement, and another muscle acts as the antagonist, relaxing and lengthening as the movement takes place. In active stretching, the extra range of movement is achieved by greater relaxation in the antagonist muscle caused by the contraction of the prime mover.

In passive stretching the player makes no contribution and does not actively contract the muscles. The movement is performed by an external agent, usually another player. Passive stretching, with a partner applying the force, requires relaxation of the antagonist muscles on the part of the player exercising and communication between the partners to ensure a safe maximum stretch without injury.

The following section gives a number of flexibility exercises which can be used either as part of the warm-up and cool-down, at either end of a training session, or as part of a planned flexibility training programme.

Flexibility exercises

Neck
1 Turn the chin in and bend the head forward gently.
2 Look up and stretch the neck back carefully.
3 Turn the head slowly from side to side.

Shoulders

4 With arms extended overhead, and with palms together, stretch the arms upwards and slightly backward (Fig 63).

5 Hold the elbow behind the head (Fig 64).

6 From the prone position stretch the arms out in front of you with fingers interlaced. Then gently lift the arms off the floor (Fig 65).

7 Adopt a 'cat stretch' position. Then, kneeling with arms out in front and with palms on the floor, press down gently (Fig 66).

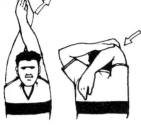

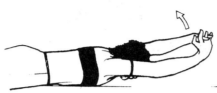

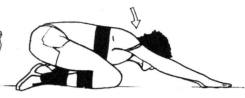

Fig 63   Fig 64   Fig 65   Fig 66

Back

8 From the prone position, place the palms of your hands on the floor by your hips and slowly and carefully raise the trunk, pushing against the floor (Fig 67).

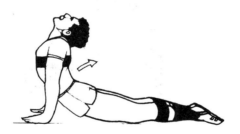

Fig 67

Gluteals and lower back

9 Lie on your back and pull one knee towards your chest with your hands, keeping the other leg straight (Fig 68).

10 From the same position, pull both knees towards the chest with your hands.

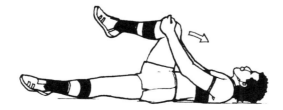

Fig 68

Hip and lower back

11 Sit and then bend your left leg at the knee and cross it over the straight right leg, resting your right elbow against the outside of your left thigh. Turn your head slowly to look over your left shoulder (Fig 69).

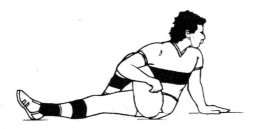

Fig 69

Hip and quadriceps

12 Place one foot forward and the other leg back with the knee almost touching the floor. Bring your hips down slowly (Fig 70).

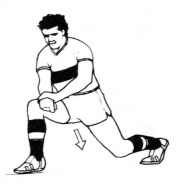

Fig 70

Quadriceps

13 From a balance on one leg, the free leg is held at the ankle with knee flexed, and the ankle is pulled carefully towards the hip (Fig 71).

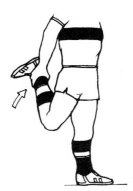

Fig 71

83

Hamstrings

14 Sit on the floor with legs together and straight. Then lift the trunk and ease it forward with the extended trunk over the legs. The hands are placed beside the feet to support the back as you lean forward (Fig 72).

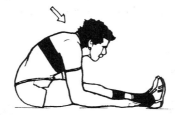

Fig 72

15 As in Fig 72, start by sitting on the floor but with one knee flexed, with your foot against the inside of the thigh of the other leg which is straight. Then lift the trunk, ease it forward, and lower the extended trunk over the straight leg.

16 The starting position is on the back with one knee flexed and the foot on the floor. The other leg is raised and clasped behind and just below the knee. Then the leg is slowly straightened, pulling the ankle back (Fig 73).

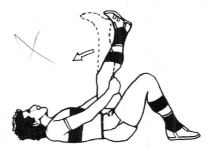

Fig 73

Groin

17 Sit on the floor with back straight and upright. The knees are flexed and the soles of the feet are put flat together. Then pull gently forward and squeeze your knees down with your elbows (Fig 74).

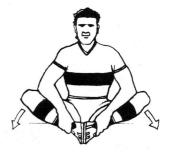

84

Fig 74

Calf

18 Lean against a solid support with the body angled back and one foot in front of the other. Keep your heels flat on the floor and gently press down over the knees until a stretch is felt (Fig 75).

19 Lean against a solid support with the body angled back and legs and feet together, standing on your toes. Your feet are placed gently flat against the floor (Fig 76).

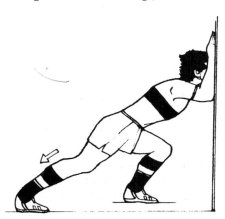
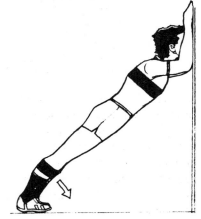

Fig 75   Fig 76

20 Adopt the front support position and rest one leg over the other. Then push the lower heel towards the ground (Fig 77).

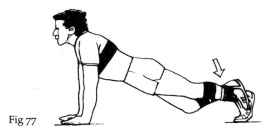

Fig 77

Ankles

21 Start sitting on the floor. Then, grasping one ankle with one hand, and hooking the knee with the elbow on the other arm, rotate the ankle slowly and gently through a complete range of motion. The foot can also be pulled gently towards the shoulder (Fig 78).

Fig 79   Fig 80

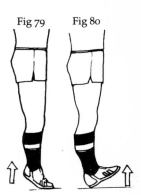

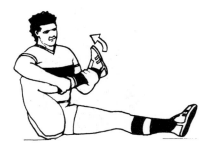

22 Standing upright, slowly raise your heels from the ground (Fig 79). Then lower the heels and raise the toes from the ground (Fig 80).

Fig 78
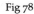

Passive static stretching

It is important that the following stretches are assisted by a sensible, careful partner and that there is good communication between the two players.

a *Shoulder stretch* (Vertical): The player sits on the ground with arms raised above his head. His partner puts his knee against the length of the player's back and gently and slowly pulls his arms backwards (Fig 81).

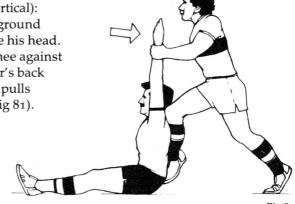

Fig 81

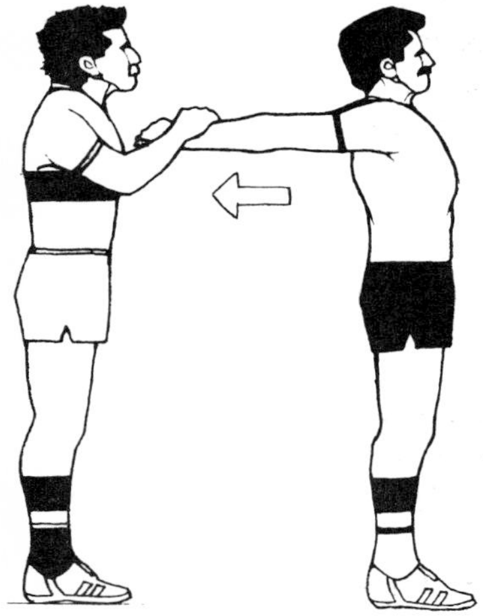

b *Shoulder stretch* (Horizontal): The player stands with his arms held out horizontally to the side. His partner takes hold of his arms and pulls them back slowly and gently (Fig 82).

Fig 82

c *Lying shoulder stretch*: The player lies on the ground face downwards with his arms out to the side. The partner stands astride the player, takes hold of his arms and carefully pulls them upwards (Fig 83).

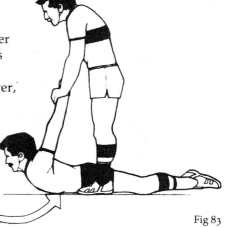

86

Fig 83

d *Abdominal stretch*: The player lies prone with his fingers interlocked behind his head. His partner stands over him and grasps his wrists and slowly pulls his trunk upwards, carefully arching the player's back (Fig 84).

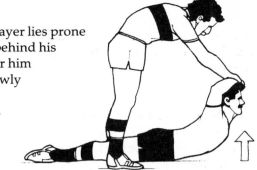

Fig 84

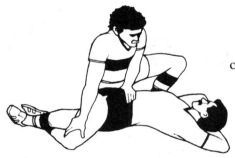

Fig 85

e *Trunk rotation*: The player lies supine with one leg across the other. The partner places one hand on his hip and carefully pushes his upper leg towards the ground (Fig 85).

f *Groin stretch*: The player sits down and puts the soles of his feet together with his heels pulled in. His partner kneels behind and presses his chest on the player's back while pressing the player's knees carefully towards the floor with his hands (Fig 86).

In an alternative exercise, both players sit upright with legs straddled and straight holding one another's wrists. One player leans forward slowly and carefully as his partner leans back a short distance (Fig 87).

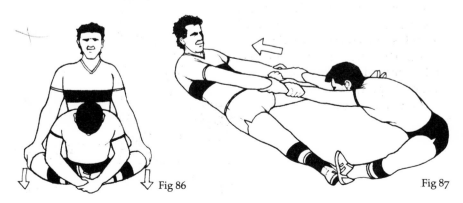

Fig 86

Fig 87

87

g *Sitting press*: The player sits on the floor with legs straight. His partner stands behind and puts his hands on the player's shoulder blades and presses carefully.

h *Hamstring stretch*: The player lies on his back while his partner, who is kneeling facing him, lifts one of his legs with the knee extended, kneeling lightly on the other leg to keep it stabilised. The partner leans against the raised leg with his shoulder (Fig 88).

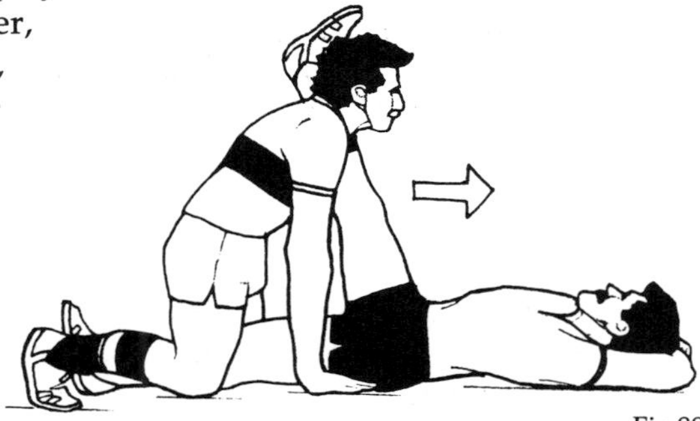

Fig 88

i *Wall press*: The player sits with his back against a wall or similar support with his legs out straight in front. His partner takes hold of both of the player's legs and presses them gently and slowly towards his head.

j *Calf stretch*: The player stands facing his partner with feet together and leans against his partner's shoulders keeping his heels on the floor. After an initial stretch, the player steps further away from his partner and repeats the stretch, keeping his body rigid and heels close to the ground.

Chapter 7

Fitness Work with the Ball

Fitness for rugby can be developed in a number of ways using the ball. This makes for the kind of practice which is directly relevant to the demands of the game because it has within it many of the game's skills. Thus, there will be some skill transfer, but it must be stressed that here the emphasis is on developing fitness using ball practices rather than on the acquisition of skill. In a session dedicated to skill acquisition a different approach would be used in the presentation, development and tempo of the practices.

These fitness practices are relatively easy to organise as they use the same equipment and facilities required for other rugby training.

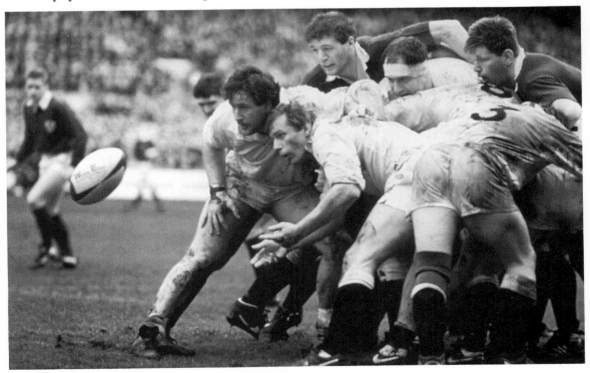

Back-row forwards Mike Teague and Peter Winterbottom feed the ball back from a controlled maul.

Warm-up/introductory practices

1 In pairs (with one ball) facing a partner, 1 metre apart: pass the ball between partners below knee and above ankle (Fig 89).

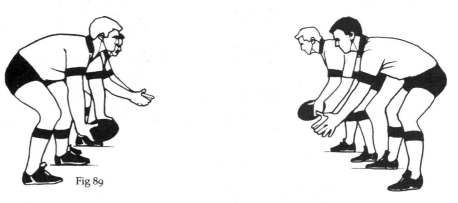

Fig 89

2 In pairs (with one ball) facing a partner, 1 metre apart in two lines: pass the ball between partners, but on a call, move 'right', 'left', 'forward', 'backwards' (Fig 90).

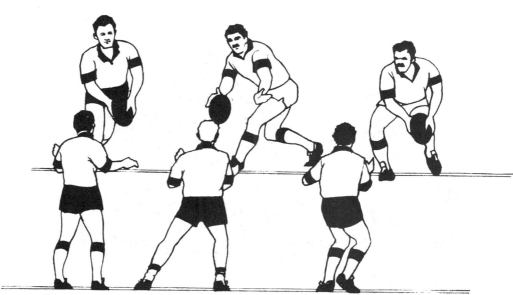

Fig 90

3 In two lines, facing each other 1 metre apart: pass the ball across, down the line. When the ball has been passed the player runs to the end of the line (Fig 91).

4 In two lines, facing each other, 1 metre apart: pass the ball along the line. When the ball has been passed, the player runs to end of the line (Fig 92).

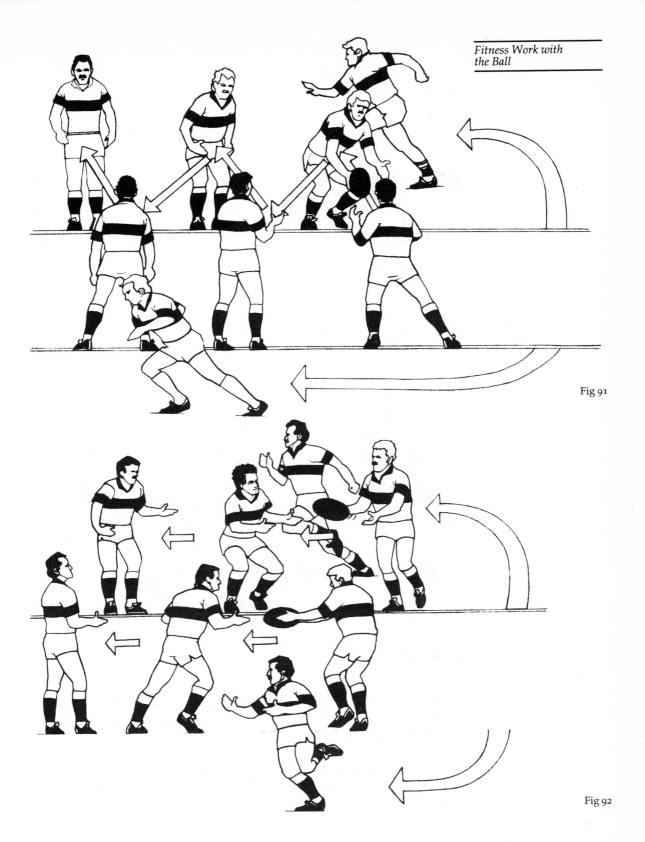

Fig 91

Fig 92

5 In two lines, running towards each other, 1 metre apart: pass the ball to the next facing player and then loop round to repeat the cycle (Fig 93).

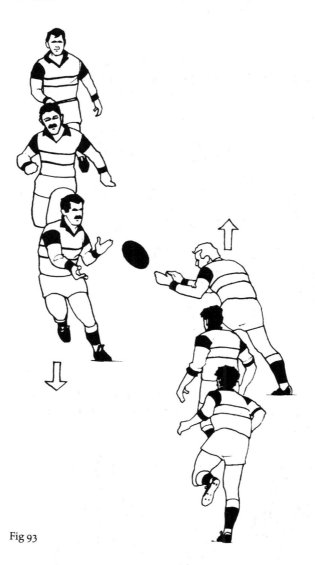

Fig 93

Using a grid

2 All players with a ball in an appropriately sized grid; run anywhere in the grid avoiding contact; on the word 'put down', players put their ball on the ground and find and pick another ball. Continue (Fig 95).

Ball familiarisation

Fig 94

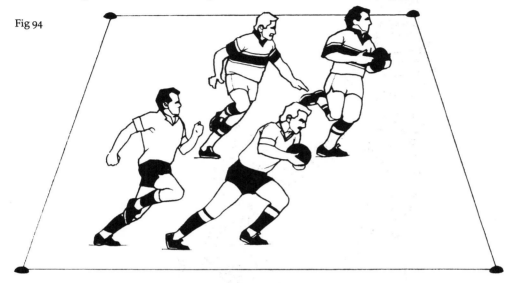

1 In pairs in a grid: with one ball between two, the player with the ball runs, dodges round the grid; his partner must follow his route exactly; then change over (Fig 94).

Fig 95

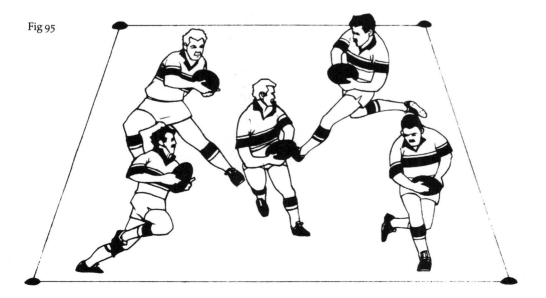

This basic practice can be developed by shouting 'On the word':
a 'Up' – the players stop and throw the ball in the air and catch it behind their backs
b 'Over' – the players stop and throw the ball from behind their backs, over their heads to catch it in front of their body
c 'Round' – the players stop and take ball quickly round their body
d 'Figure-of-Eight' – the players stop and take ball round and through their legs in a figure-of-eight movement
e 'Kick' – the players on the move kick the ball a short distance in the air to catch and then continue running.

These calls can be given at random to maintain alertness and concentration.

3 Players in pairs with one ball between them; moving anywhere in the grid, passing the ball quickly between themselves (Fig 96).

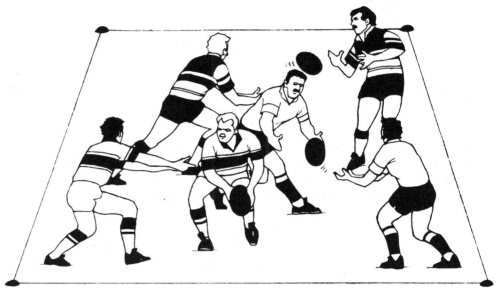

Fig 96

This basic practice can be developed by shouting 'On the word':
a 'Down' – one player places the ball on the floor for his partner to pick up on the move
b 'Kick' – one player grubber-kicks the ball along the floor for his partner to pick up on the move
c 'Up' – one player throws the ball in the air for his partner to jump and catch
d 'Set' – one player moves ahead with the ball, turns to face his partner who drives in, takes ball, and rolls off to continue running.

3 v. 1, keep ball

Three players move around the grid, and keep the ball from the one in opposition (Fig 97)

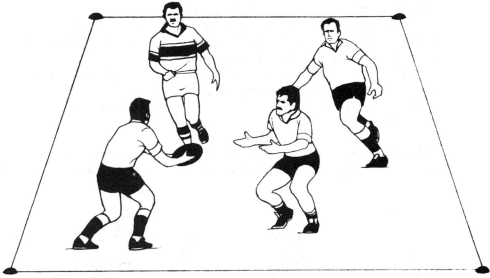

Fig 97

2 v. 2, keep ball

Two players move around the grid, and keep the ball from the two opponents: contact can be introduced by allowing the opposition to make a standing tackle on the ball carrier who must remain on his feet and place the ball on the floor with two hands to be released (Fig 98).

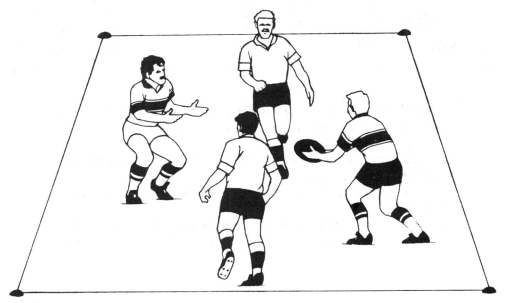

Fig 98

Crossover

Players line up at corners of the grid. As each player arrives at the front of the line, he runs across the grid and passes the ball to the first player opposite him (Fig 99).

Two balls can be used at first, then four balls, one for each group. This basic practice pattern can be developed in the following ways:

1 The receiving player can anticipate the pass and run forward to receive it.

2 The ball can be placed on the ground for the receiver to pick up.

3 The player runs straight through but makes his pass to the group on the left.

4 The player runs straight through but makes his pass to the group on the right.

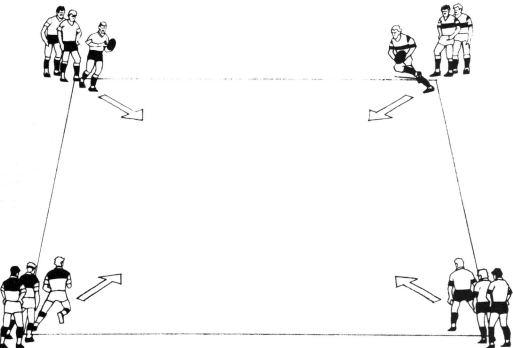

Fig 99

5 The player runs across the grid, passes the ball to the first player opposite him and then chases him back across the grid trying to touch him on the back.

6 Players can run to any corner which is free and has no other player running towards it.

7 Bring the four groups closer together so that there is less space available to cross in the middle of the grid.

8 Players line up in six groups. The same practices can be repeated but with six groups (Fig 100).

9 Corner groups run across as shown but the players in the middle groups can go to left or right depending from which side they received the ball. They will run to the corner from which they received the ball.

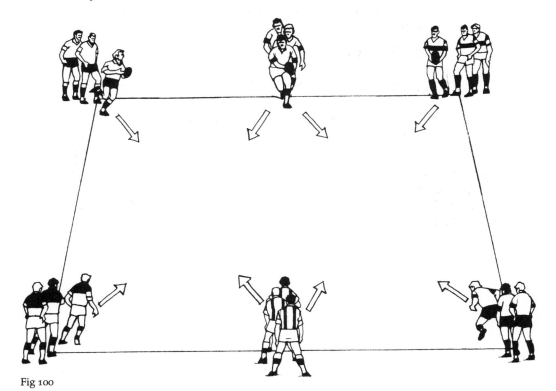

Fig 100

Shuttle running

Shuttle running is a useful method for improving a player's anaerobic capacity and speed endurance. This work can also include a ball.

1 In pairs, the front player with a ball; he sprints to a line 15m away and places ball on the ground, sprints back to the original line and then back to pick up the ball. Repeat for 30 seconds. Thirty seconds work; 30 seconds rest. Alternate with partner. 5 to 8 repetitions (Fig 101).

Fig 101

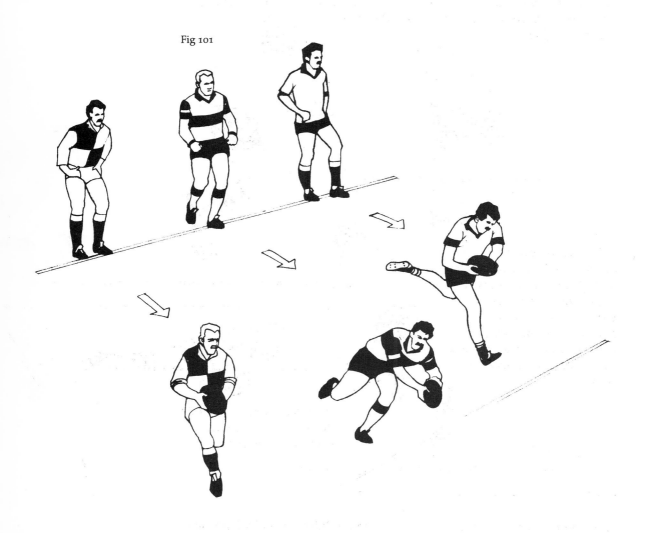

2 This basic practice pattern can be developed in the following ways:

a In two lines, 10m and 15m, the same practice, carrying the ball and putting it on the 15m-line but running 'double shuttles' to 10 and 15m. As before, 30 seconds work: 30 seconds rest. Alternate with partner. 5 to 8 repetitions.

b In three lines, 5m, 10m and 15m, the same practice carrying the ball and putting it on the 15m line but running 'triple shuttles' to 5m, 10m and 15m. As before, 30 seconds work, 30 seconds rest. Alternate with partner, 5 to 8 repetitions.

c Partner stands on a line 10m away, facing the player holding the ball. Player sprints out, takes the pass, runs on to the 15m line, turns back, gives the ball back to partner on his way back to the original line. thirty seconds work, 30 seconds rest. Alternate with partner. 5 to 8 repetitions (Fig 102).

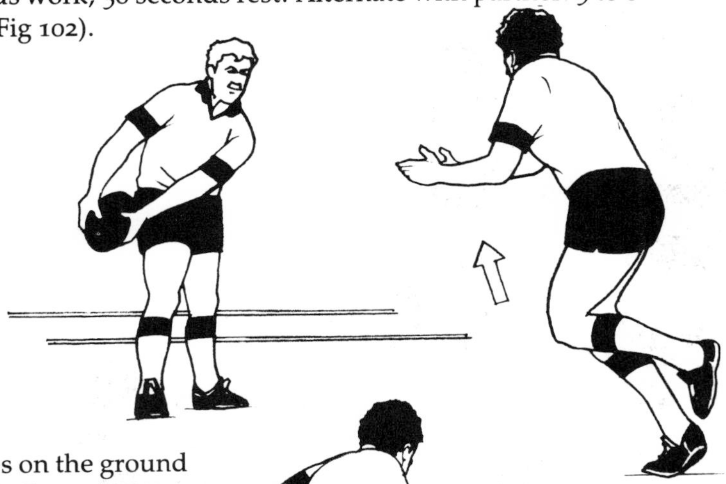

Fig 102

d Partner lies on the ground around the ball on a line 10m away from the player who sprints out, steps over partner, takes the ball and sprints on to the 15m line, turns and gives the ball back to his partner on his way back.

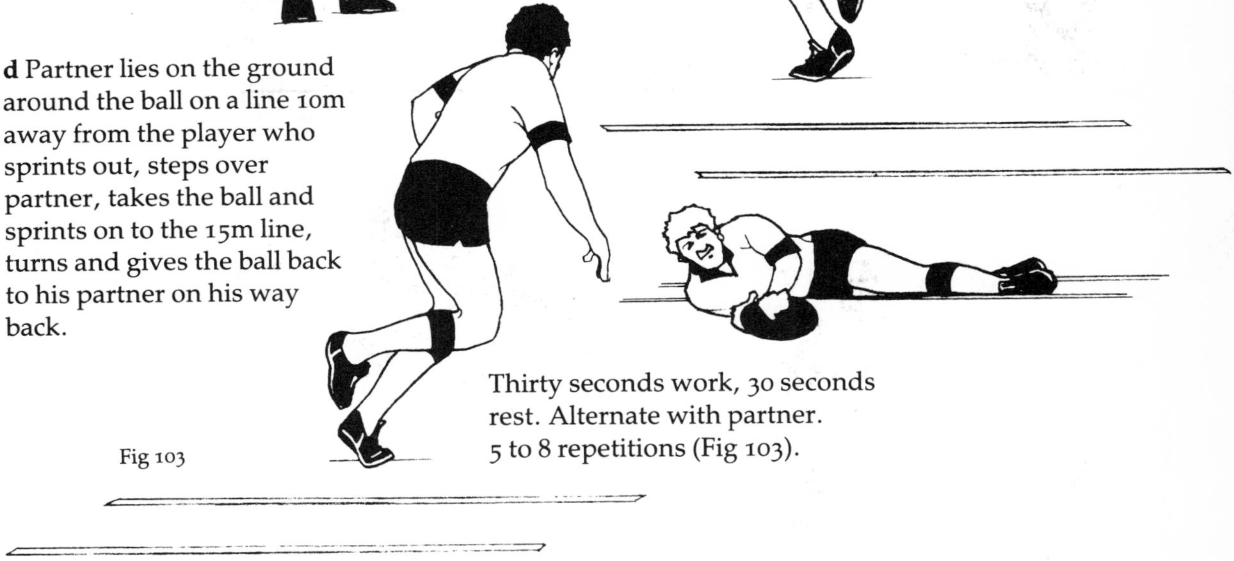

Thirty seconds work, 30 seconds rest. Alternate with partner. 5 to 8 repetitions (Fig 103).

Fig 103

The intensity of these practices can be increased/decreased by lengthening/reducing the work interval or increasing/reducing the number of repetitions.

'Rob the nest'

Six rugby balls in the middle. When a number is called, that player from each team races to take the balls one at a time and place them in his own 'nest'. When the nest of footballs in the centre has been exhausted he may rob any other team's nest, taking one ball at a time. The first team to gain three balls wins (Fig 104).

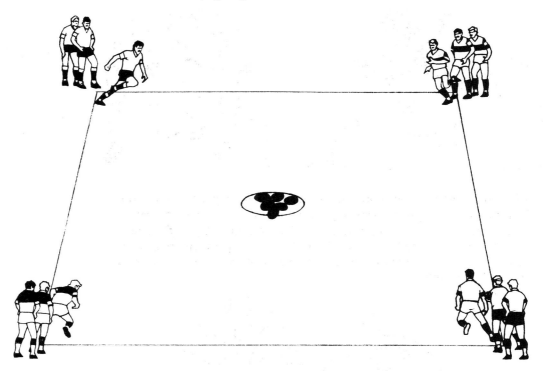

Fig 104

Strength/power work

1 One ball between two players, one holds ball, his partner tries to get hands on ball and 'rip it away' from the player in possession. Change round (Fig 105). After each session of 'wrestling' for the ball, the two players bind together, adopt a low body position, sprint to a line 10 metres away and run back (Fig 106).

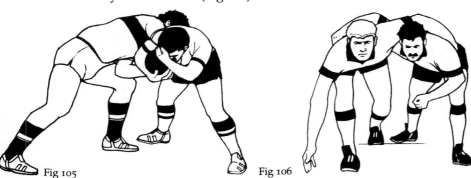

Fig 105   Fig 106

2 One ball between four players. Two partners have possession of the ball, the two in opposition try to get their hands on the ball and 'rip it away' from the players in possession. Change round (Fig 107). After each session of 'wrestling' for the ball, the four players bind together in a line, adopt a low body position and run to a line 10 metres away and run back (Fig 108).

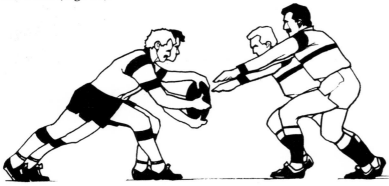

Fig 107

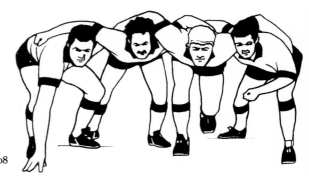

Fig 108

Chapter 8

Body Composition, Nutrition and Diet

'The trouble with Italian food is that six days later you're hungry again'
(Marathon runner Frank Miller)

Body composition

Because rugby football is a contact game the size and weight of a player is important. While basic body shape can be altered only slightly, substantial changes can be made in a player's body composition, that is, the proportion of body fat to lean body weight.

Lean body weight refers to all body tissue which is not fat, for example, muscle, bone and body organs. With rugby players in training, any changes in weight will result primarily from changes in the balance between fat and muscle mass, so any changes in lean body weight will reflect changes in muscle mass.

Energy balance

The aim of every player must be to have a greater proportion of 'lean' weight and a lower proportion of 'fat' weight contributing to his total body weight. In order to achieve this it is necessary for calorific expenditure to match (or exceed) calorific intake; this is the basic concept of energy balance. By energy, we mean the capacity to perform work.

Although the concept of energy is a complex one, in simple terms the human body converts chemical energy, found in the foodstuffs and drink we consume, into mechanical or kinetic energy. Mechanical work can be performed by, for example, jumping in the line-out, driving forward in the scrum and sprinting with the ball. All energy associated with movement is kinetic energy.

A player is in energy balance when the amount of energy taken in by the body equals the amount of energy expended by the body. When intake exceeds output, the excess energy is stored as fat or wasted in some way. If the intake of energy does not meet the body's energy demands, then the additional energy needed will be taken from the body's fat stores.

Nutrition

The aim of good nutrition is to provide sufficient energy for the demands of training and matches while at the same time maintaining, or improving, the proportions of lean body weight to body fat.

It would be true to say that for the most part we eat and drink without much thought and understandably assume that our bodily requirements will be met. We all enjoy eating socially and our choice of food is therefore based on 'eating for entertainment' rather than 'eating for energy'. However, the rugby player in serious training has to ensure that his training and match-demands are being optimally met by his diet; if they are not, how should his diet be modified?

A good diet makes its greatest impact by helping to support the recovery period between training sessions. Improvements in fitness, as we have already said, are the result of the body adapting to the stress of intensive training, adaptations which require the intake of necessary nutrients. Occasional indulgences in diet are of no consequence but it is important to pay attention to eating habits 365 days of the year – not simply on the few days prior to matches.

The energy demands of training

All forms of training increase the body's need for energy; and the more demanding the training, the greater is the energy requirement.

Energy is mainly derived from the carbohydrate and fat in food and, to a lesser extent, protein. Once the carbohydrate is consumed it appears in the blood as glucose. This can then be used directly for energy or stored in the muscle, or in the liver, as glycogen, an important source of energy for the rugby player. A limited amount – about 200g (7oz) – can also be stored in the muscles. On the other hand, we store energy more abundantly in our bodies as fat. An adult rugby player may have 14kg (30lb) of fat in his body stored in many places – under the skin, around vital organs and among muscle fibres.

During a training session and during a match, the working muscles derive much of their energy from the glycogen stored within the muscles and liver. The muscles can, and do, get energy from the fat deposits in the body but when a player is training or playing intensively his energy requirement is so great, and needed so rapidly, that only carbohydrates can produce the energy fast enough. Only a small proportion of fat would, therefore, be used at this level of effort.

The harder the training or the work during a game, the more dependent is the player on his supplies of carbohydrates – the glycogen stores. In fact, the glycogen stored in the muscle probably determines the amount of work which can be done by that muscle. Consequently, the diet should be high in carbohydrates with approximately 50 to 60 per cent of the total energy intake coming from that source.

The need for carbohydrates

The best high-carbohydrate foods are those in which the carbohydrate exists in the natural, unrefined state; for example, in wholemeal bread or brown bread; in wholemeal flour for all baked goods – pizzas, pastries and biscuits; in breakfast cereals that contain the whole grain of the wheat, unpolished rice, wholemeal spaghetti and pastas. This means eating fresh or frozen vegetables (particularly root and green leafy vegetables), potatoes (especially baked in the skins), fresh and dried fruit, beans and peas. These and other similar types of food are high in carbohydrate, fibre, vitamins and minerals while being relatively low in energy: they are only fattening when large amounts of fat are added.

Complex carbohydrates

Bread consumption may be increased but in making sandwiches it is essential to reduce the amount of butter and margarine. When trying to increase the carbohydrate intake, emphasis must be placed on what are called complex carbohydrates (wholemeal bread, potatoes, peas, baked beans, cereals, fresh fruit – apples, bananas and oranges – and dried fruit – apricots and prunes). There should be limited reliance on confectionery or sweet foods (the sugars or simple carbohydrates) to provide the dietary carbohydrate. The day should be started with a breakfast which is high in complex carbohydrates, such as muesli or wholegrain cereals, and fresh fruit juice, tea or coffee.

The overall amount of fat in the diet should be reduced. This means reducing all the visible fat (butter, lard, oils, fat on meat) and non-visible fat (milk, dairy produce, eggs, mayonnaise, sausages, paté, pies and pastry). There is no need to eat large amounts of red meat. Instead of the high-fat meats, such as lamb, beef, pork and duck, there should be an emphasis on lean or white meats – chicken, turkey, and so on. Similarly, white fish should replace the oily fish, such as mackerel or tuna.

The consumption of fried foods should be reduced, with emphasis on grilling, stir-frying or steaming. Any fat which appears during cooking should be poured off. Adding fat to a dish, for example in the form of gravy, sauces, butter to hot toast or on baked potatoes, should be avoided. Alternatives to mayonnaise or oil-based dressings for salads should be tried – natural yoghurt or citrus fruit juices can be used on their own or as a basis for dressings.

Diet and general health

This emphasis on increasing the amount of carbohydrates in the diet and reducing the amount of fat makes sense in terms of general health as it agrees with recent recommendations for healthy eating. These suggest that more carbohydrates should be introduced so that they provide half or more of the energy in the diet. At the same time less fat should be consumed, especially fats of animal origin. There is, therefore, no conflict between eating for training and eating for health – the approach is to concentrate on carbohydrate-rich foods at most meals.

Present evidence on protein intake indicates that the normal dietary intake of about one gram of protein per kilogram of body weight is sufficient for rugby players in training. This will meet any increased requirement (say, for a player on a strength training programme) so long as the total energy intake is adequate to maintain body weight.

Increasing the amount of protein in the diet or consuming large amounts of protein supplements is unlikely to have any beneficial effect. Protein consumed in excess of requirements will be used simply as a source of energy, stored as fat or excreted from the body. Also eating high-protein foods and large amounts of meat and dairy produce will leave little appetite for the necessary high-carbohydrate foods.

The best approach is to enjoy a high-carbohydrate diet. This will provide necessary energy and keep the glycogen stores full during training in addition to the normal intake of protein which is present in a varied and balanced diet.

Fluid balance

One important dietary factor when training is the fluid balance. Our bodies consist of about 70 per cent water; thus, in a 70kg player, 49kg is water. Fluid balance or hydration is of prime importance to the rugby player in training, as even a slight reduction in body water can cause a reduced efficiency in cellular function. Dehydration also deprives the body of sufficient water to cool itself and so the body may overheat, particularly in warm training or playing conditions. Thirst is a poor indicator of the need to start taking fluids. The need is to ensure that you maintain a high fluid intake by drinking plenty of water and fresh fruit juice as part of a normal diet. It is essential to be fully hydrated before training sessions. This means taking water about half an hour before training and small amounts of fluid, when appropriate, from time to time during the training session. Unfortunately, any drink containing alcohol causes extra urinary loss of water. As it acts as a diuretic, it should be avoided as an aid to fluid balance.

Organising the player's diet

Many rugby players lead a pretty full life so it is often sensible eating which suffers in the total training programme. It is important that a player organises himself so that he eats enough to 'refuel' between training sessions and matches. It is useful to eat carbohydrates directly after training sessions and matches in order to refuel the carbohydrate stores in the body; there is evidence that intake at this time has the best impact. If breakfast is missed then it is wise to include a good mid-morning snack. Before evening training, it is a good idea to eat something around 3 or 4 p.m. and to have the main meal after training. Appetite will probably increase as the volume and intensity of training increase. Here the aim is to eat more carbohydrates, but not to overeat. Rest days are important – to give the body time to recover from the stresses of training. This extra time should be used to eat sensibly to make up for any hurried meals eaten on training days and to refuel carbohydrate stores.

The following section illustrates the eating habits recommended for a rugby footballer and shows different examples of meals which may be eaten for breakfast, lunch, dinner or snacks at home. These meals are nutritionally balanced and are high in carbohydrate. The portion sizes are intended as guidelines and may vary according to your personal tastes (28g is equivalent to 1 oz).

A high-carbohydrate low-fat diet for rugby players

Breakfasts		
	Cornflakes – 80g Skimmed milk – 400ml Banana (chopped) – 100g Sugar – as required Fruit juice – 250ml	Bread/toast – 2 slices Low-fat spread – 10g Jam, honey, marmalade or marmite
	Weetabix – 60g Muesli – 30g Skimmed milk – 450ml Banana – 100g Sugar – as required	Fruit juice – 250ml Crumpets – 80g Low-fat spread – 10g Jam, honey, marmalade or marmite
	Branflakes – 60g Raisins – 30g Skimmed milk – 400ml Banana – 100g Sugar – as required	Fruit juice – 250ml 2 tea cakes – 100g Low-fat spread – 10g Jam, honey or marmalade
	Fruit 'n' fibre – 80g Skimmed milk – 400ml Banana – 100g Sugar – as required Fruit juice – 250ml	Bread/toast – 2 slices Low-fat spread – 10g Jam, honey, marmalade or marmite
	Shredded Wheat – 60g Raisins – 30g Skimmed milk – 400ml Banana – 100g	Fruit juice – 250ml Malt loaf – 60g Low-fat spread – 15g

	Porridge/Ready Brek – 70g
	   raw weight
	Raisins/Sultanas 30g
	Skimmed milk – 400ml
	Golden syrup – 20g
	Fruit juice – 250ml
		Bread/toast – 2 slices
		Low-fat spread – 15g
		Jam, honey, marmalade or
		   marmite

Lunches

Bread – 4 slices
Low-fat spread – 20g
1 egg (hard boiled)
Lean ham – 60g
	Salad (tomato, lettuce,
	   cucumber, celery,
	   watercress)
	Doughnut
	Banana – 100g

6 crumpets – 240g Low-fat spread – 30g Low-fat cheese – 40g (Shape, Tendale, '15%') Marmite	2 fruit scones – 100g Jam, honey or marmalade Pear
2 large pitta bread – 180g Tuna in brine – 150g (drained weight) Salad	Salad cream/dressing Doughnut Low-fat yoghurt – 1 carton
Oxtail/lentil/vegetable soup – 400g Bread/toast – 2 slices French bread – 150g	Low-fat spread – 30g Low-fat cheese – 40g Salad Apple
Bread – 3 slices Low-fat cheese – 25g Low-fat spread – 20g Banana	Baked beans – 225g 2 tea cakes (toasted) – 100g Jam, honey or marmalade
Bread – 3 slices 2 bread rolls 1 egg (hard boiled) Low-fat yoghurt – 1 carton	Canned spaghetti – 225g Low-fat spread – 20g Salad Orange

Dinners

Potatoes (boiled, baked, mashed or microwaved) – 300g
Low-fat spread – 10g
Lean gammon steaks – 20g
Tinned pineapple – as required
Peas – 150g
Rice pudding (low-fat brand or homemade with
   skimmed milk) – 400g

Spaghetti – 100g (raw weight)
Bolognese sauce (made with lean minced beef) – 200g
Mixed vegetables – 150g
Fruit salad – 200g
Low-fat yoghurt – 1 carton

Potatoes – 300g
Chicken piece (skin removed – grilled, baked, boiled or
    microwaved) – 150g
Boiled broccoli – 150g
Baked beans – 225g
Fruit pie filling – 225g
Custard (made with skimmed milk) if required

Macaroni – 100g raw weight
Packet cheese sauce
Tuna in brine – 150g (drained weight)
Tomato
Prunes – 200g
Custard if required

Rice – 100g (raw weight)
Curried beans – 400g
Mixed vegetables – 150g
Tinned mandarin oranges – 300g
Low-fat yoghurt – 1 carton

Potatoes – 300g
Low-fat cheese – 30g
Turkey breast (boiled, baked or microwaved) – 150g
Peas – 100g
Tomato
Rice pudding (low-fat brand) – 400g

Snacks   Bread/toast – 3 slices
Baked beans/canned spaghetti – 400g
Breakfast cereal – 60g
Skimmed milk – 350ml
Raisins – 25g
Sugar if required

Rice pudding (low-fat brand) – 400g
Piece of fruit

Bread – 3 slices
Low-fat spread – 20g
Jam, honey, marmalade or marmite
Low-fat yoghurt – 1 carton

Malt loaf – 80g
Low-fat spread – 20g
Piece of fruit

Canned ravioli – 400g
Bread – 3 slices

Snacks may be taken regularly throughout the day to increase carbohydrate intake and to maintain total energy intake while on a diet lower in fat. Some carbohydrate should be consumed as soon as possible after training to speed glycogen resynthesis and to aid recovery. Examples of convenient snacks to carry around include:

> Pieces of fruit
> Sandwiches
> Currant buns
> Scones
> Malt loaf
> Drinks

Fluids should be taken regularly throughout the day; drinks that are high in carbohydrate include:

> Fruit juices
> Squashes
> Soft drinks
> 'Sports drinks', such as Lucozade or Gatorade

Other drinks which contain carbohydrate plus useful amounts of nutrients include:

> Build-up (made using skimmed milk)
> Complan   ,,
> Ovaltine   ,,
> Low-fat Horlicks   ,,

Eating out

Many players have a lifestyle which often necessitates them eating out or having a quick snack out. Suggestions are given in the following section for snacks which can be prepared at home and carried around and a few guidelines as to the choice of food in restaurants:

Snack meals

> Cartons of skimmed milk, fruit juices and cans of diet drinks
> Fresh fruit – bananas, oranges, pears, apples, grapes, melon, and so on
> Dried fruit – apricots, raisins, dates, tropical fruit mix
> Canned fruit (unsweetened)
> Canned rice pudding (preferably the low-fat variety)
> Low-fat flavoured/plain yoghurts (with added muesli, packed separately)

Wholemeal bread rolls, pitta bread, wholemeal bread, brown french bread, wholegrain crispbread with any of the following fillings:

> tuna (canned in brine or water)
> salmon, prawns (fresh or canned)
> sardines, pilchards (canned in tomato sauce)
> low-fat cottage cheese
> low-fat cheese spreads
> reduced-fat cheese (small amounts) (for example, Edam, Tendale, reduced-fat Cheddar type)
> turkey, chicken (grilled, roast or steamed at home or bought cooked)
> lean red meat: ham, beef, pork (with all visible fat removed)
> boiled egg with reduced-calorie mayonnaise

and/or

beetroot and other pickles	reduced calorie coleslaw/mayonnaise
shredded white cabbage	beansprouts
lettuce	grated carrot
cucumber	tomatoes
sweetcorn	cress
mushrooms	green/red/yellow peppers
onion	kidney beans
mixed pasta salad (without oily or creamy dressing)	mixed rice salad (preferably brown)

So a few suggested snack meals from the above are:

> Wholegrain pitta bread with brown rice salad and salad vegetables, one hard-boiled egg, fruit yoghurt and orange juice.
> Sardine and salad roll (no need for butter or margarine), mixed bean salad with pasta shells, apple, nuts and raisins.
> Wholemeal bread roll (hoagie-type) with lean beef, low-calorie coleslaw, mustard, tomato and cucumber, orange.

Choice of food in cafes/restaurants

Try not to choose dishes:

> cooked in fat or oil
> coated in breadcrumbs/batter/fried in oil
> in thick, creamy sauces
> in pastry

Try to choose: wholemeal bread and bread rolls (go easy on butter or margarine)
fresh fruit without ice-cream/cream for dessert, and fruit sorbets in preference to ice-cream.

Type of restaurant	Try to choose	Try to avoid
Pizza	Wholemeal vegetarian pizza. Seafood pizza	high-fat toppings, salami, olives, cheeses
Hamburger	Hamburger with salad. Fruit juices	Cheeseburger, baconburger, chips, thick shakes
Italian	Pasta with meatless sauce, such as marinara or vegetable. Tossed salad (without oily dressing)	Pasta with cream, butter or oil-based sauces, Italian sausage
Chinese	Stir-fried chicken, seafood, vegetables and steamed rice. Fruit sorbet	Deep-fried in batter fried rice. Dishes with cream, butter, or oil-based sauces
Indian	Mixed grills, seafood or chicken dishes without creamy sauces. Vegetables and steamed rice. Fruit sorbet	Deep-fried in batter, fried rice, dishes with cream, butter or oil-based sauces

Pre-match eating

There are many misconceptions about pre-match eating. The ability to perform heavy and intensive exercise during the match is directly related to the initial glycogen stores in your muscles. When you run on to the field, if glycogen stores are low, the capacity to maintain a high work-rate for 80 minutes will be impaired. How you have eaten during the days prior to the game can have an influence on your performance. It is necessary to have an adequate intake of carbohydrate in preparation for the match. So the week leading up to the game and particularly the last two days should see an increased carbohydrate intake.

However, this does not mean that the player should cram in food during those two days. There should be a gradual increase in carbohydrate and fluid throughout the week with no heavy meals. This means

111

smaller, more frequent high carbohydrate meals which are easier on the stomach. Last-minute stock-piling is harmful rather than helpful so, for example, the meal of Friday evening should be relatively light.

Although fluid intake is important and must be maintained it does make good sense to avoid alcohol in the 24 hours before kick-off.

Match day

Any meal on match days should be taken 3 to 4 hours before kick-off to allow plenty of time for digestion. One important reason for this is that the player needs a good blood supply to the muscles to produce energy during the match. The digestive system also requires a blood supply; thus eating a meal causes extra blood to flow to the digestive system. If the meal comes too close to the game there is competition between stomach and muscles for the available blood supply. Anxiety will also tend to slow down the rate at which food moves through the system.

The meal on match days should be light, easily digestible and consist mainly of carbohydrates. It is a matter of finding out what works best for the individual, because personal preference is important. Match day is not the time to try something new, so the aim must be to eat food to which the body is accustomed and which suits individual digestions.

Certain myths still abound such as the pre-match steak, which is not at all beneficial and can be harmful. The time needed to digest a steak, and other fatty meats, is considerable (12 to 18 hours). This means, almost certainly, that only limited energy would be released from such a meal. Fat in any form should be kept to a minimum in this pre-match period, as it slows down the emptying time from the stomach.

Some players are in the habit of taking glucose drinks or tablets before a game. Such supplements can help energy production but the effects are short-lived. They can also affect adversely the release of glycogen from the muscles which is the important and substantial source of energy from carbohydrates. Thus, it is important not to take excess amounts – never more than 50g in any hour.

Once you have eaten, try to relax, as rushing around will also slow down digestion. And try to avoid any last-minute snacks. After the match, try to eat some carbohydrate food as soon as possible in order to start to build up the carbohydrate stores again.

Chapter 9

Fitness Testing

'My doctor told me that jogging would add ten years to my life.
He was right. I feel ten years older already'
(Milton Berle)

Since physical fitness is a major factor in every player's match performance, a game provides a rough, if subjective, way of assessing and
evaluating a fitness training programme. In addition, physical and physiological parameters can be measured at various stages of the programme in order to monitor the training-induced changes in the player's
fitness. The results of these tests can also be used to provide a form of
'fitness profile' for each player which will highlight his strengths and
weaknesses.

In order to assess training-induced changes in fitness or to identify a
player's strengths and weaknesses, it is important to appreciate that
fitness for a game such as rugby football is not only multi-dimensional but
also varies according to the player's position on the field.

So, having identified the fitness demands of the game, the requirement
is to identify fitness tests which measure the components of fitness
highlighted in the match analysis. The tests themselves should also be
viewed as a means to an end – to plan individual training programmes
based on a player's strengths and weaknesses. At the same time, the tests
do help players to understand more about themselves from a fitness point
of view and provide the rationale for their fitness training schedules.

The following are among the more important components of fitness for
rugby:

> Body composition
> Aerobic endurance
> Flexibility
> Speed and acceleration
> Upper body muscular endurance
> Leg power
> Anaerobic capacity

In the following section these qualities will be explained with the outline
of an appropriate test.

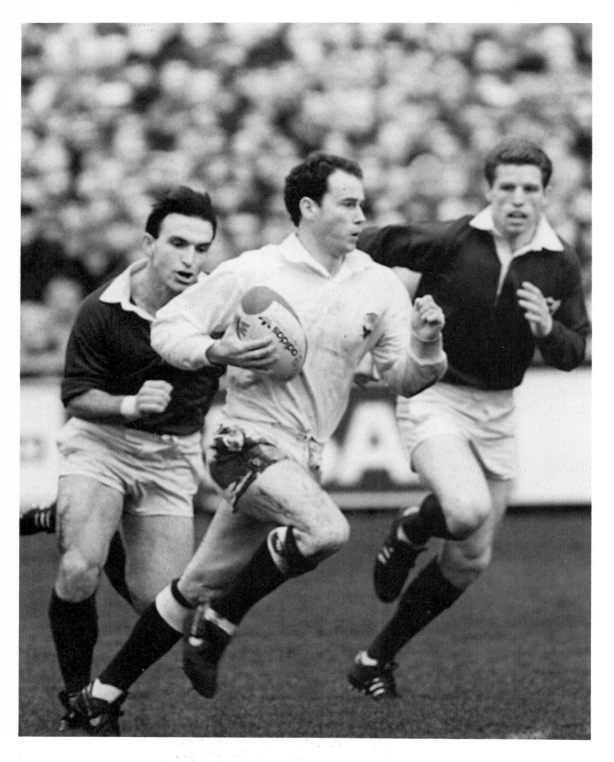

England full-back Simon Hodgkinson employs both pace and swerve
to take on Ireland's Dave Curtis and Brendan Mullin on the outside.

Body composition

In addition to measurements of height and weight, skinfold thickness can be taken to record the body composition of the player. In simple terms, the body may be regarded as being composed of two 'compartments' – body fat and lean body mass (muscle, bones and organs). Together they make up the total body weight. It is the proportion of body fat to lean body mass (that is, our body composition) that is more important than our actual body weight, since changes in body composition may occur without a change in body weight. In other words, an increase in muscle mass may be accompanied by a similar decrease in body fat resulting in no change in body weight. In addition, an increase in body weight may occur if the increase in muscle mass exceeds the loss in body fat. Body composition measurements, therefore, may be more informative than the change in overall body weight.

In general, body fat accounts for 15 per cent of the total body weight of males and 25 per cent of females, and these figures are usually lower for men and women actively engaged in sport. In physical activity, such as rugby football, where body weight is carried, excess body fat may be detrimental to performance. This is because body fat represents 'dead weight' that has to be carried around the field. On the other hand, because of the physical nature of the game, certain playing positions may require slightly higher proportions of fat than others, in order to protect the vital body organs in contact situations.

Test

Standard measurements of weight and height can be taken for each player. Skinfold thicknesses can be measured at four sites on the body (triceps, biceps, subscapular and iliac crest) and used in conjunction with approved methods for the calculation and estimation of body fat and lean body mass (Fig 109).

Equipment: Skinfold calipers, measuring tape.

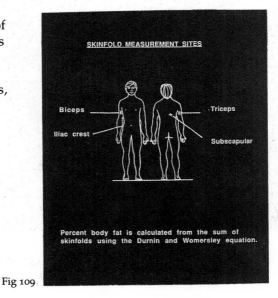

SKINFOLD MEASUREMENT SITES

Biceps — Triceps

Iliac crest

Subscapular

Percent body fat is calculated from the sum of skinfolds using the Durnin and Womersley equation.

Fig 109

Fig 110

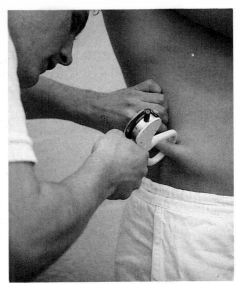

Method:
The skinfold is picked up between thumb and forefinger and pulled slightly away from the underlying tissues. The caliper jaws are applied immediately below the finger and thumb. The measurement should be read on the calipers after the full pressure of the jaws has been applied which is two seconds after release of the trigger (Fig 110).

Skinfold thicknesses can be measured on:

1 Triceps – with the arm hanging vertically relaxed, midway between the tip of the acromion process and the olecranon process
2 Biceps – with the arm resting supinated, over the belly of the muscle, at the same level as the triceps
3 Subscapular – under the inferior angle of the scapula, the fold pointing slightly downwards and outwards
4 Iliac crest – 1 cm above the iliac crest at the side of the body with the fold running forwards and downwards.

Aerobic endurance

A good indicator of a player's endurance capacity is the measurement of 'maximum oxygen intake'. This is the highest amount of oxygen that a player can transport from the air to the working muscles. It is one of the factors which dictates the work rate a player can achieve at various stages of the game, and over the full 80 minutes, as it influences energy output to an important extent.

There is an obvious advantage in achieving a high level of endurance fitness when players are running continuously and have also to maintain a high work rate throughout the game, especially during the final quarter when fatigue creeps in. However, endurance fitness is also important for players involved in brief periods of highly intense activity because fitness in this area leads to a faster recovery. For example, a winger might be involved in a series of sprints with little recovery between each, or a prop might be involved in an important scrum just after having sprinted across the pitch.

Test

The test involves the indirect determination of maximum oxygen intake. A 20m shuttle-run test is used to determine indirectly each player's maximum oxygen uptake ($\dot{V}O_2$max). The test involves running 20m shuttles at speeds dictated by a sound signal emitted from a cassette recorder. Approximately every minute the speed of the shuttle is increased. The aim of the test is to keep pace with the sound signal for as long as possible. The point at which the player can no longer keep up with the required pace is recorded and used to estimate $\dot{V}O_2$max. For example, if a player reaches level 12 or 13 he will have a predicted $\dot{V}O_2$max of between 54.3 to 57.6ml/kg × minute respectively.

(Multi-stage test tapes are available from the National Coaching Foundation, 4 College Close, Beckett Park, Leeds.)

Flexibility

Flexibility is probably the most neglected and undervalued component of physical fitness. Lack of flexibility can cause poor performance and inefficient technique as well as being a possible underlying cause of many of the strain and tear-type injuries in rugby football. Poor flexibility can also hinder speed and endurance since the muscle has to work harder to overcome resistance. By increasing the possible range of movement, especially in the lower body, the player can exert force over a greater range of movement, thus increasing his power. In addition, if the player can increase his flexibility to provide for a greater range of movement than is actually required in the game this is an effective means of injury prevention.

A range of flexibility tests can be used but two possible measures are:

Test

Sit and reach test: This measures hamstring and lower back flexibility. After some warm-up stretches the player adopts a long-sit position, legs straight, with the soles of his feet placed against a 'sit and reach' board. He places his hands on the measuring surface and stretches forward, gently pushing the wooden baton as far as the stretch allows (Fig 111). The distance is then measured from his feet, a positive score if the baton is past his feet and a negative score if he is unable to reach his toes. A modified test can then be performed on each leg separately in order to show any imbalance in flexibility between the two legs. While one leg is being tested the other will be gently flexed and supinated.

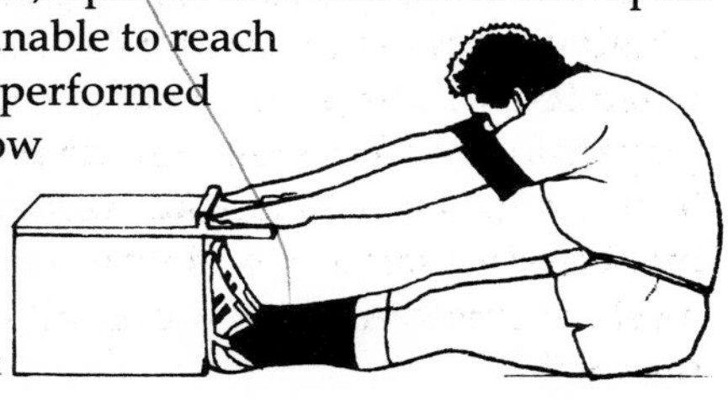

Fig 111

117

Dynamic flexibility: A dynamic test can be used to assess upper body mobility and flexibility. The player stands with his feet a shoulder width apart and is required to touch, alternately, a cross on the floor in front of him and a cross at shoulder height on the wall behind him as many times as possible in 20 seconds (Fig 112).

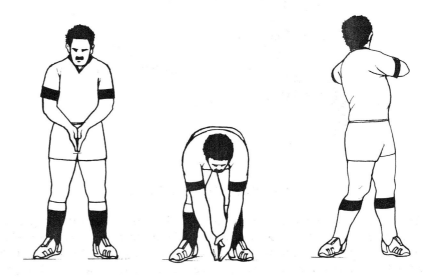

Fig 112

Speed and acceleration

An important fitness requirement of the rugby player is the ability to accelerate quickly from either a stationary or moving start in addition to achieving the fastest possible running speed. Although this is an obvious quality in certain positions, the wings for example, it is particularly valuable to a team if all players can increase their basic running speed, particularly over shorter distances.

Test There are difficulties associated with accurate timing, particularly over shorter distances, when using a hand-held stop-watch, because of problems with human error and false starts. Also the improvement in times for a short sprint is very small and in repeated tests the equipment needs to be sensitive enough to record accurately the slight changes which occur. Testing speed, therefore, requires simple electronic timing, using the beam of a photo-electric cell. Any distance from 5m to 50m can be selected and the player starts 1 metre behind the first beam. Timing will begin once the first beam has been broken and will be stopped when the player crosses the beam of the finish line (Fig 113).

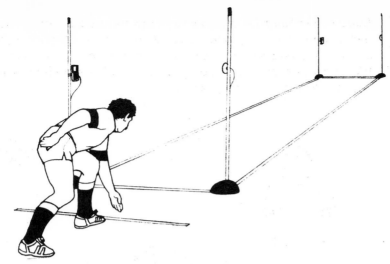

Fig 113

Muscular endurance

In addition to aerobic endurance and the need to develop general 'runnability', the player also needs muscular endurance which represents the capacity for continuous performance of relatively heavy localised activity which may make only small demands on the functions of respiration and circulation before exhaustion sets in. This type of endurance is essential in rugby football, especially in the arm, shoulder and abdominal regions.

Tests

For abdominals

Paced trunk curls. This test will be performed with bent legs, feet supported and arms folded across the chest, hands resting on opposite shoulders. The test will be at a standard pace. The players have to stay in rhythm with a series of bleeps on an audio-cassette (for example, 50bpm) by touching elbows to thighs on one bleep and then touching their shoulders to the floor on the next (Fig 114). Each player does as many trunk curls as possible until he loses form. Losing form will include

    1 not touching elbows to thighs
    2 moving the hands from the shoulders
    3 inability to maintain pace with the bleeps
    4 bouncing.

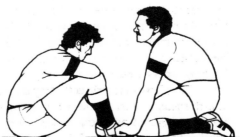

Fig 114

119

For arm and shoulders *Paced push-ups*. This test is also performed to a series of bleeps on an audio-cassette (for example, 50bpm). Players perform an 'extended' push-up which involves the muscle groups of the chest as well as those of the arms and shoulders. In order to standardise the placement of hands, players first lie on the gym mat in a prone position, with arms out to the side and elbows flexed at 90 degrees. The position of the elbows determines where the hands will be placed for the performance of the test. Players start with the arms extended and feet together. On the first bleep they move to a flexed arm position with their chest touching the tester's clenched fist, placed on the mat immediately under their chest. At the next bleep players should be in the extended position with straight arms (Fig 115). The player does as many push-ups as possible until he loses form. Losing form will include:

 1 not touching chest to the fist
 2 not extending the arms fully
 3 bending or sagging at the hips
 4 inability to maintain
  pace with the bleeps.

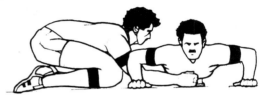

Fig 115

Strength and power

The importance of developing the strength and power component of fitness is obvious in a game like rugby football. However, the specific strength requirements within the game may vary considerably including strength endurance, explosive strength, static strength, maximal strength and power. While some strength gains may result from general fitness training, specific gains in strength will be dependent on the type of training being undertaken and the muscle groups being used. It is important to appreciate that to improve one aspect of strength, such as explosive strength, requires different training methods from those required to improve strength endurance. Consequently, the strength training requirements may vary considerably between the playing positions in the squad or team.

Test Because of the varied strength and power qualities required in the game, a range of strength tests could be used, but one obvious quality for all players, particularly the forwards, is leg power.

A good and more accurate alternative to the Sargent Jump test is the use of a jump meter. The meter is fixed round the waist of the player with the end of the cord attached to a rubber mat on which the player stands. With any necessary arm swings the player bends at the knees and drives vertically upwards from the mat (Fig 116). The height of the vertical jump is recorded on the meter.

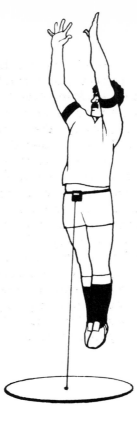

Fig 116

Anaerobic capacity

The ability to produce a high power output for a short period of time is essential for the rugby player. However, unlike the sprinter who performs one bout of maximal exercise and then may not compete again that day, a rugby player is required to reproduce continual bursts of high intensity exercise and be able to cope with the consequences of such effort – namely the production of lactic acid. Rugby football can thus be termed a 'multiple-sprint activity'. Consequently, fitness for rugby football, in terms of anaerobic performance or sprint performance, is not based on the ability of a player to produce one maximal sprint but to be able to keep reproducing fast sprints or short bouts of high intensity work. A good anaerobic capacity for this type of work will help a player to maintain high power outputs over relatively long periods, or alternatively to keep bursts of activity with a minimal loss of power.

Tests

The test is designed to provide an estimation of speed endurance based on a fatigue index.

Each player is required to sprint at maximum speed over a 40m shuttle, with a 20-seconds recovery period between sprints. The time for each shuttle sprint is recorded by hand, using a stop-watch.

121

Test procedure:
1 A player starts with his feet behind the centre line.
2 He sprints to the end line (10m), turns and sprints to the far end line (20m), turns and sprints to the centre line (10m): total 40m.
3 Maximal effort is required for all sprints: no pacing.

Table 14

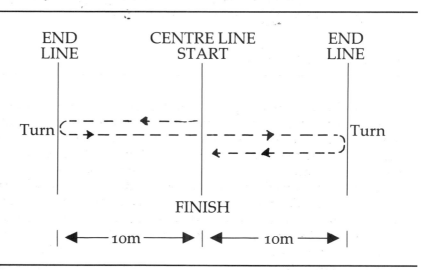

Fatigue index: A fatigue index, used to assess a player's speed endurance, is calculated by taking the average of his two fastest sprints away from the average of the two slowest sprints. The time difference between the two fastest and the two slowest sprints is then expressed as a percentage of the two fastest sprints. The percentage decrease in time between the two fastest and the two slowest sprints can be expressed by this formula:

$$(T7 + T8/2) - (T1 + T2/2) = D$$
$$D/(T1 + T2/2) \times 100 = x\%$$

where T1 & T2 = the two fastest sprints
    D = Difference
    T7 & T8 = the two slowest sprints
    X% = % drop in pace

In a club situation it may be simpler to calculate the fatigue index by subtracting the fastest time recorded from the slowest time, that is, 9.1 seconds (slowest) − 8.1 (fastest) = 1.0 (fatigue factor).

Table 15 Example calculation of Fatigue Index

	Sprint
1	8.66
2	8.59
3	8.74
4	8.73
5	8.70
6	8.98
7	8.88
8	8.95

1. Mean of two slowest times minus mean of two fastest times:

$$\frac{8.98 + 8.95}{2} - \frac{8.66 + 8.59}{2} = 0.34$$

2. Difference between fastest and slowest divided by the mean of the two fastest as a percentage:

$$\frac{0.34 \times 100}{8.62} = 3.94\%$$

Fatigue Index = 3.9%

The testing of international players

The senior England rugby squads are tested on a regular basis throughout the year in order to monitor their fitness development, to provide a fitness profile for each player, and to evaluate the effectiveness of their fitness training programme. The programme of fitness tests described in the previous pages are the ones used with the England players.

As already explained, the main purpose of fitness testing is to provide guidance for the planning of the players' individual training programmes which will be based on their strengths and weaknesses. As international rugby players they are also set targets on each test. Three categories have been established: 'élite', 'very good' and 'acceptable'. For the speed and acceleration tests the targets have been governed by the playing positions of the team. The following Table 16 shows the targets for each test.

Table 16 Fitness test targets

Body fat			
	Elite	Sub. 12%	
	Acceptable	Sub. 15%	
V̇O₂max. test			
	Elite	65ml/kg/min.	(15/4)
	Very good	60ml/kg/min.	(13/11)
	Acceptable	55ml/kg/min.	(12/6)

15m sprint (seconds)	*Front five*	*Back row/ Hooker*	*Backs*
Elite	sub. 2.40	sub. 2.30	sub. 2.20
Very good	sub. 2.50	sub. 2.40	sub. 2.30
Acceptable	sub. 2.60	sub. 2.50	sub. 2.40

30m sprint (seconds)	*Front five*	*Back row/ Hooker*	*Backs*
Elite	sub. 4.30	sub. 4.20	sub. 4.00
Very good	sub. 4.40	sub. 4.30	sub. 4.10
Acceptable	sub. 4.50	sub. 4.40	sub. 4.20

Trunk curls		**Push-ups**	
Elite	125+	Elite	70+
Very good	100+	Very good	55+
Acceptable	75+	Acceptable	40+

Leg power

Elite	75cm+
Very good	65cm+
Acceptable	55cm+

Sit and reach

Elite	20cm+
Very good	15cm+
Acceptable	10cm+

England players have been fitness tested since 1988 and there has been continual improvement in their tested performances, reflecting an increase in the fitness levels of the squad. The following Table 17 shows the average values for the England forwards, the backs and the whole squad in some of the tests.

Table 17 Average values for England players on a selection of tests

	Body fat %	Endurance $\dot{V}O_2max$ ml/kg × min	Flexi-bility cm	Muscular endurance		Leg power cm	Speed and acceleration	
				Trunk curls	Push-ups		15m sprint (s)	30m sprint (s)
Forwards	15.4	56.7	11	101	53	56	2.50	4.34
Backs	11.7	60.0	12	101	48	66	2.12	3.86
Squad	13.7	58.2	12	101	51	60	2.38	4.13

Glossary

Adenosine triphosphate [ATP]. High energy chemical compound which is formed with the energy released from food and is stored in all cells, particularly muscle cells. Used as energy supply for muscle and other body functions; the energy currency

Aerobic. In the presence of oxygen; aerobic metabolism utilises oxygen

Anaerobic. In the absence of oxygen; non-oxidative metabolism

Antagonist muscle. The name given to muscle or muscles which cause the opposite action to that produced by agonist (prime movers)

Body composition. Refers to the proportions of lean body mass and body fat

Calorie. A unit of work or energy equal to the amount of heat required to raise the temperature of one gram of water one degree centigrade

Capillaries. Small vessels in a fine network located between arteries and veins where oxygen, food and hormones are delivered to tissues and carbon dioxide and waste products are picked up

Carbohydrate. A chemical compound containing carbon, hydrogen and oxygen. Carbohydrates are one of the basic foodstuffs used for energy and are stored in the muscle and liver as glycogen

Creatine phosphate. A chemical compound which is stored in the muscle and when broken down helps to manufacture ATP

Connective tissue. Material found in many tissues, especially muscle, consisting largely of collagen. It is relatively strong and resistant to stretching and provides strength and structure for tissues such as tendons and ligaments

Eccentric contraction. Muscular contraction in which the muscle lengthens while developing tension

Energy. The capacity to perform work

Enzyme. A protein compound which speeds up chemical reactions

Fat. A foodstuff containing glycerol and fatty acids. An important energy source, stored for future use when excess fat, carbohydrate or protein is ingested

Fatigue. Diminished work capacity. A state of tiredness, discomfort and decreased efficiency resulting from prolonged or excessive exertion

Glucose. A form of sugar and an energy source transported in the bloodstream.

Glycogen. The form in which glucose is stored in muscles and the liver. It is the primary carbohydrate storage form in animals

Glycolysis. The breakdown of glycogen to lactic acid

Heart Rate (HR). The number of times the heart beats per minute

Hydration. The restoration of normal fluid reserves of the body

Isokinetic. Muscular contraction against a resistance which is varied to maintain high tension throughout the range of movement while speed remains constant

Isometric. Muscular contraction in which tension is developed but with no change in the length of muscle; contraction against an immovable resistance

Kinetic energy. Energy associated with motion and movement

Lactic acid. A by-product of anaerobic glycolysis resulting from the incomplete breakdown of carbohydrates

Ligament. A band of sheet-like fibrous tissue connecting bones

Maximum oxygen uptake ($\dot{V}O_2$max). The maximum rate at which oxygen can be consumed per minute; the power or capacity of the aerobic system

Metabolic rate. The sum total of the chemical changes or reactions occurring in the body

Muscle spindle. A proprioceptor (sense organ which gives information concerning movements and positions of the body) located within special fibres called intrafusal fibres

Obesity. Excessive body fat

Overload. Exercising a muscle or group of muscles against a resistance greater than that which is normally encountered

Phosphocreatine system. (see Creatine phosphate)

Power. The rate of doing work (work per unit of time); if one kilogram is raised one metre in one second, power is expressed as one kilogram-metre per second

Prime mover. Name given to a muscle or muscles which are directly responsible for producing or controlling a specified joint action

Protein. An organic compound formed from amino acids; a basic foodstuff which forms muscle tissues, hormones, enzymes and so on

Recruitment. The process by which skeletal muscle fibres are stimulated to contract and participate in the generation of force

Repetition maximum (RM). The maximum load a muscle or group of muscles can lift in a given number of repetitions before

fatiguing. For example, a 5-RM is the maximum load that can be lifted 5 times

Resistance. Any force that impedes movement

Respiratory system. The uptake of energy from the atmosphere into the lungs and then via the blood to the tissues and exhalation of carbon dioxide from the tissues to the atmosphere

Set. A unit containing a fixed number of repetitions

Skinfold. A pinch of skin and subcutaneous fat from which total body fat can be estimated

Tendon. A band of fibrous tissue forming the termination of a muscle and attaching the muscle to the bone

Twitch. A single contraction induced by electrical stimulation of skeletal muscle fibres

Vitamin. Organic nutrient in the presence of which metabolic reactions occur

Further Reading

Bob Anderson, *Stretching* (Pelham, 1981)
Rex Hazeldine, *Fitness for Sport* (Crowood, 1985)
Rex Hazeldine, *Strength Training for Sport* (Crowood, 1990)
Radcliffe and Farentinos, *Plyometrics: Explosive Power Training* (Human Kinetics, 1984)
Steve Wootton, *Nutrition for Sport* (Simon and Schuster, 1988)

INDEX